The Real Truth About
WOMEN
and
AIDS

How to Eliminate the Risks
Without Giving Up
Love and Sex

Helen Singer Kaplan, M.D., Ph.D.

Director, Human Sexuality Program
The New York Hospital–Cornell Medical Center

A FIRESIDE BOOK
Published by SIMON & SCHUSTER, Inc.
NEW YORK • LONDON • TORONTO • SYDNEY • TOKYO

10 9 8 7 6 5 4 3

Library of Congress Cataloging in Publication Data

Kaplan, Helen Singer
    The real truth about women and AIDS.

    "A Fireside book."
    1. AIDS (Disease)—Popular works. 2. Women—Diseases. 3. Safe sex in AIDS prevention. I. Title.
    [DNLM: 1. Acquired Immunodeficiency Syndrome—popular works.
    2. Women—popular works.
    WD 308 K17r]
    RC607.A26K37 1987   616.97'92   87-23504
    ISBN 0-671-65783-6
        0-671-65743-7 Pbk.

This publication is intended to provide accurate information with regard to the present understanding of the subject matter covered. Every individual's health needs are unique and dependent upon that individual's circumstances. The publisher does not intend this book to provide individuals with medical advice, which should properly be provided by a physician or qualified health professional.

The author is grateful to the following for permission to reprint:

Figure 2. "Patients with AIDS and Carriers," from "Shadow on the Land: The Epidemiology of HIV Infection," by Drs. Robert R. Redfield and Donald S. Burke, in *The American Journal of Immunology.* Copyright © 1986 by *The American Journal of Immunology.* Reprinted by permission.

Table 3. "Homosexual Behavior Patterns," from *Homosexualities.* Copyright © 1978 by Alan P. Bell and Martin S. Weinberg. Reprinted by permission of Simon & Schuster, Inc.

Figure 4. Data on county-specific prevalence of HIV infection in civilian applicants for military service from October 1985 to March 1986 from "Shadow on the Land" by Drs. Robert R. Redfield and Donald S. Burke, *The American Journal of Immunology,* copyright © 1987. Reprinted by permission.

"When to Test for AIDS," Editorial in *The New York Times,* May 17, 1987. Copyright © 1987 by The New York Times Company. Reprinted by permission.

"The A.C.L.U.'s Myopic Stand on AIDS," Op-Ed by Charles Rembar, in *The New York Times,* May 15, 1987. Copyright © by The New York Times Company. Reprinted by permission.

"On AIDS and Moral Duty," Op-Ed by Willard Gaylin, in *The New York Times,* April 24, 1987. Copyright © 1987 by The New York Times Company. Reprinted by permission.

"Second AIDS Tests Increase Accuracy Dramatically," Letter to the Editor by Michael Marmor, in *The New York Times,* May 23, 1987. Copyright © 1987 by The New York Times Company. Reprinted by permission.

To Jennifer

Contents

Consultants

1. *Stephen Udem, M.D., Ph.D.*—Associate Professor, Department of Medicine, Division of Infectious Diseases, Albert Einstein College of Medicine.

2. *Michael Marmor, Ph.D.*—Associate Professor, Department of Environmental Medicine, New York University Medical Center Testing, Epidemiology.

3. *Phillip Kaplan, M.D.*—Postgraduate Fellow, New York University, Department of Pathology.

Why I Hate to Talk About AIDS

For the last twenty-five years I have loved helping people with sexual problems and conducting research to improve theories and methods of sexual therapy. It is a joyful experience for me to help free a patient from a sexual disability that has cast a cloud over his or her life, or to see a couple's marriage improve as they begin to overcome their long-standing sexual difficulties. I love telling people: "Enjoy, it's okay to have sexual feelings . . . Sex is a natural function . . . Sex is not dirty or harmful . . . Don't give your kids sexual hangups!"

But now I find myself warning people, especially our young women: "Look out! Sex with an infected partner is dangerous." I hate to be negative about sex. I feel bad, like I used to when I had to restrict my children's spontaneity and sternly warn them not to run across the street: "You can't go until the light is green, until you look left and right, until you are *sure* that you are safe — the traffic can kill you." And now I hear myself saying: "You can't have a full sexual experience with anyone until you are *sure* that you and your partner are not infected — AIDS can kill you."

I would much rather talk about the joys of sex and love and intimacy, but I feel doctors and scientists must speak up about the dangers of sex, *now!*

I was born in Vienna and am a refugee from the Holocaust. I have long been troubled by the thought that if voices had been raised in protest early on, if someone had warned us in the early 1930s at the first sign of the Nazi plague, *before* the fascists became firmly entrenched, perhaps the tragedy of the mass exterminations could have been prevented. We can't go back to that time, but it is still early enough to prevent a general AIDS *epidemic.* Fortunately, AIDS has not *yet* become firmly entrenched in the general population. We still have time and we have the means and the technology to prevent a tragedy that could exterminate more people than the Holocaust did!

I have never written a book for the public before, but I have interrupted my main work of teaching, research, publishing scientific texts, and treating patients to write this book because I feel that the American people, especially women, are being victimized by inaccurate information and misleading "educational" programs which have grown out of the political struggle surrounding AIDS, and that *it is still not too late to prevent a major disaster.*

I will try to tell you what you need to know without political bias and distortion. My only aim is to help you protect yourself and your unborn children. But I will try to show you that you can do this without sacrificing your sex life or your romantic relationships. *You do not have to choose between life and love.*

I have made every effort to distinguish known facts from good educated guesses, from pure theory, and from downright lies. But remember, *new information about AIDS is accumulating so rapidly that what is written here today may have changed by tomorrow.* Therefore, remember that the advice and suggestions I have made in this book are well founded on current scientific information, but in a developing situation like this, nothing said comes with a guarantee, nor could it.

1

Why a Book for Women? Myths and Facts

I have addressed this book to women because women are the next group expected to become infected with AIDS.

You are extremely vulnerable, but the urgent need to protect you and your children is being neglected by the public health and the political establishments.

You hear: "Don't get hysterical, nothing is going to happen to you" and "Relax, just use a condom . . . Forget it, you'll be okay."

That is exactly how I heard my parents and their friends talk, when the Nuremberg Laws were first passed: "Relax, Hitler is crazy, he'll be gone by next year, just sit it out."

That is just what we heard six years ago, when the first AIDS cases were noted: "Don't be an alarmist, don't talk about a plague, it's just happening to a few gay men."

But look at the world's experience with AIDS! Look at Africa, where the disease is widespread and affects both men and women equally. Now thousands are dying of the

Table 1   *AIDS in Men and Women: Increase in Heterosexual Transmission to Women Between 1983 and 1986*

	WOMEN	MEN	TOTAL	% FEMALE	% FEMALES INFECTED THROUGH SEXUAL CONTACT
1983	162	2213	2375	6.8%	(14%)
1984	302	4384	4686	6.4%	(17%)
1985	569	8062	8631	6.6%	(20%)
1986*	729	9775	10504	6.9%	(26%)

* Cases reported through Nov. 7, 1986.
Source: Guinan, M. E., and Hardy, A. Epidemiology of AIDS in Women in the United States. JAMA 1987; 257: 2039.

This chart depicts a dramatic change in the way women contract AIDS. Through 1986, most women who became infected did so through contaminated drug needles, but now, sex with an infected man is the main danger for women.†

disease and a substantial number of babies born to women carriers are doomed to a tragic death in infancy!

On the other hand, Cuba has protected women and their offspring. All Cubans who were assigned to Angola, in Africa, must be tested upon their return, and those who became AIDS carriers are confined in hospitals in order to "avoid (sexual) transmission," and so far no infections have been reported in women or children.‡

Many experts are predicting that there will be a massive AIDS epidemic like the bubonic plague that wiped out one-third of Europe more than 600 years ago. It is impossible to say if this will prove true, but there are enough alarming indications that this fatal disease is about to spread in epidemic proportions to the general population that we simply cannot afford to take any chances.

There is little doubt that women will be the next victims of the oncoming epidemic. Already, the rate of sexual transmission of HIV (AIDS) to women has doubled. You must protect yourself. You need to know the true facts about AIDS in order to survive.

† Personal communication with Dr. Mary E. Guinan.
‡ According to the April 17, 1987, edition of *Garma*, an English-language newspaper published in Cuba, there are now 108 carriers of the AIDS virus confined to hospitals. Three male patients have died of AIDS.

It is shocking to me to read and hear the false alarms, false reassurances, half-truths, distortions, misleading information, and outright lies that are being dispersed through the media, by some of the so-called "sex education" programs, AIDS hotlines, and counseling services. Even the recent how-to-avoid-AIDS books that I have seen are not telling the whole truth about AIDS.

MYTHS AND TRUE FACTS

Let's examine some of the common myths about AIDS, and you will see just how confusing and dangerous to your health such misinformation can be.

1. **Myth:** There is no danger of AIDS infection if you always use condoms.

   Fact: Latex condoms (not lamb) reduce the risks, but the level of protection is not known. There is no doubt however, that you *can* get AIDS if you have sex with an infected man who uses a condom *even if it does not break.*

2. **Myth:** An AIDS carrier does not really have AIDS, so he cannot infect you.

   Fact: A carrier can most certainly give you AIDS if you have sex with him or receive his blood. Carriers are called "healthy" only because they have no outward signs or symptoms of AIDS, but they are infected with and harbor the HIV (AIDS) virus in their body fluids. *Carriers are contagious,* presumably for life.

3. **Myth:** The AIDS virus is transmitted only through sex and blood.

Fact: AIDS can be transmitted through sex, through all infected body fluids, and through pregnancy. Women carriers very likely will give birth to AIDS babies, many of whom will be dead before they reach two years of age.

4. **Myth:** You cannot get AIDS from oral sex.

Fact: It is possible to become infected through any sexual act that involves the mingling of your body fluids with those of an AIDS carrier. Therefore any "wet sex," that is, anal sex, vaginal sex, oral sex (both him to her and her to him), and possibly also wet kissing, is *not safe if your partner is infected.*

5. **Myth:** The only way to avoid getting AIDS is to give up all sex unless you are in a long-term monogamous relationship.

Fact: Monogamy with a partner who is known to be free of HIV (AIDS) infection is certainly one way to eliminate the risks. But there are also many perfectly safe "dry" sexual practices which you can enjoy with partners whose AIDS status you are not sure of.

6. **Myth:** AIDS testing is not necessary to prevent the spread of AIDS.

Fact: AIDS testing is considered *essential* for protecting women because "healthy" carriers can be detected only with the AIDS antibody test, and women can avoid sexual exposure and eliminate the risks of infection only if they know the AIDS status of their partner. With AIDS, *what you don't know can kill you!*

7. **Myth:** Exposure is the same thing as infection.

Fact: Exposure and infection are completely different. You have been *exposed* if you have had sexual contact with an infected person, while *infection* means that the virus has invaded your body. The only people who need to be tested are those who have been exposed to AIDS. Then they can know if they have actually been *infected*.

8. **Myth:** Testing should not be done because it is not cost-effective.

   Fact: It costs less than $3.00 for each ELISA AIDS screening test. The confirmatory Western blot test is more expensive, about $7.50, but seldom necessary because the majority of low-risk heterosexuals will be negative and the Western blot test is only used to confirm positive results. Compared to the $50,000 to $150,000 and more that it costs to provide medical care for a single patient with AIDS, *testing is extremely cost-effective.*

9. **Myth:** Adolescents should not be tested because very few are infected.

   Fact: Do not confuse *low prevalence* with *low risk*. Low prevalence refers to the *current* rate of infection. Low risk means that persons of that group are not likely to *become* infected in the future. Adolescents have a *low prevalence* of AIDS but a *high risk* of being infected in the near future. It is precisely because they are still largely uninfected but are clearly in danger that adolescents, especially those in inner cities, should be protected by testing.

10. **Myth:** A single exposure is not dangerous. You have nothing to worry about unless you have had multiple sexual partners and have been exposed many times.

    Fact: Several women have become infected from a *single exposure* to an infected man and even from one artificial insemination with semen from an infected sperm donor.* The risks do go up with each exposure, but you *can* get AIDS from one sexual experierice with an AIDS carrier.

11. **Myth:** So many men are infected now that you can not avoid exposure to the AIDS virus if you want to have sex.

Fact: In the country as a whole only one out of every thirty thousand† drug-free heterosexual men is infected today, and these men are referred to as "low-risk" men. Up to 70 percent of male homosexuals, I.V. drug users, and hemophiliacs are infected in some areas of the country and make up the "high-risk" groups.‡

12. **Myth:** Chances that any man you might meet and go to bed with has AIDS are probably less than one in thirty thousand.

Fact: That is true if he is "straight" and from Montana, but if he is a bisexual from a place like New York, the chances rise to as high as seven in ten (70 percent).

13. **Myth:** Do not be alarmed, there is no AIDS epidemic, only gays have to worry.

Fact: Be alarmed! The number of women who have gotten ill with AIDS by way of heterosexual transmis-

---

* Scientific References, Group VI, Heterosexual Transmission of AIDS.

   Because of the highly technical nature of the documentation, I have referenced groups of sources on a particular topic rather than footnoted individual articles. In order not to interrupt the reader I have used these sparingly throughout the book.

† These estimates are based on blood bank studies for the entire country. The risk is probably significantly higher than 0.003 percent in "high-risk" areas like New York City, San Francisco, and Washington, D.C., and lower in "low-risk" rural areas.

‡ Scientific References, Group I, The Epidemiology of AIDS.

sion has *doubled* in the past year and is continuing to rise at a frightening rate. While the number of American women who have been infected with AIDS is still small, less than 0.01 percent in the country as a whole, experts believe that women are directly in the path of the oncoming epidemic.

14. **Myth:** All the body fluids of AIDS carriers are infected, so you should not use bathrooms, telephones, or eating utensils that homosexuals have used.

Fact: AIDS, like syphilis, gonorrhea, and genital herpes, is a *sexually transmitted disease*, and you do not get ill from eating with or socializing with a person who has those conditions.

SEXUALLY ACTIVE WOMEN ARE NEXT

It is a common misconception that AIDS is still exclusively a "gay" disease. While 75 percent of AIDS cases in this country have occurred in male homosexuals, it has been estimated that 27 percent of males who are infected with the AIDS virus are heterosexually active bisexuals or I. V. drug abusers.* This is very dangerous because the virus is increasingly being transmitted through heterosexual contact to women and adolescents.

Sexually active American women who live ordinary lives, who work, who go to school, women of all social classes, are increasingly at risk for the following reasons:

1. *Heterosexual Transmission to Women Is Increasing Rapidly.*

Until recently, heterosexual transmission accounted for only a small fraction (1 percent) of AIDS infections. This

* Scientific References, Group I: The Epidemiology of AIDS.

means that today most women who have AIDS got ill from using a contaminated needle to inject themselves with narcotics or because they were given a contaminated blood transfusion. The chances that a woman got AIDS from an infected sexual partner are still extremely remote. Presently, in 1987, 99.9 percent of American women are still uninfected, and females make up less than 7 percent of the AIDS cases that have been reported to the U.S. Centers for Disease Control in Atlanta.

This seems trivial. Nothing to worry about. But there are alarming indications that AIDS is in the process of breaking out from the highly infected gay and drug-user groups, among whom it reached epidemic proportions in the last four years. AIDS *is beginning to move into the general population.* AIDS has already appeared in increasing numbers of female prostitutes from "high-risk cities": these women have been heavily exposed because many use intravenous drugs, and also because they have casual sexual contact with many high-risk males (see Figure 1 in Chapter 2 for the distribution of AIDS in the U.S.), and the majority of women who are married to or are the steady sexual partners of known AIDS carriers, mostly intravenous drug abusers or bisexuals, are already infected!

Table 2   *AIDS Infection in Female Prostitutes by Geographic Area*

The CDC report of seroprevalence in U.S. prostitutes is based on 568 study participants for whom HIV antibody status was determined. This was a multicenter study including women from seven distinct areas of the country. The geographic region and seroprevalence found are as follows:

1. Newark/ Jersey City/ Paterson	57.1%
2. Miami	18.7%
3. San Francisco	6.2%
4. L.A.	4.3%
5. Colorado Spgs	1.4%
6. Atlanta	1%
7. Las Vegas	0.0%

Source: Antibody to HIV in Female Prostitutes. MMWR 1987; 36: 157.

AIDS is just beginning to spread to women and their babies and to adolescent girls. If we act NOW, if we get women to "hear" the truth about AIDS, and to protect themselves, and if we act in unison and pressure our politicians to put programs into effect that are specifically designed for the protection of women, we can nip this epidemic in the bud. It is not too late!

2. More Men Than Women Are Infected.

Despite the age-old adage that women are the transmitters of venereal diseases, with AIDS it seems to be the other way around. At this time in the United States for every woman who is infected with AIDS virus, there are approximately 15 infected men. So, the ratio of males with AIDS to females with AIDS is approximately 15 to 1. Assuming that the ratio of HIV carriers parallels the ratio of AIDS cases, by sheer mathematics the chances of an American man giving the disease to an American woman are much greater than that of a man catching it from his female partner. To put it another way, if male-to-female transmission and female-to-male transmission were equally probable, for every 15 women who would get AIDS from making love to an infected man, only 1 man would get it from an infected woman.

It is also possible that the infection passes more easily from a man to a woman than from a woman to a man. We have learned from studying the homosexual transmission of AIDS that the *receiver* of semen in anal sex is more likely to become infected than the *emitter*, and it had been thought that the transfer of semen to the woman's body during vaginal intercourse makes it more likely for the female partner to become infected. But some of the newer studies are suggesting that male-to-female and female-to-male transmission may be occurring with equal frequency. That is what seems to be happening in Africa. There are several good studies now under way comparing the male-to-female and female-to-male transmission rates, and we will understand this better soon.

The AIDS epidemic is spreading at a geometric rate. That means very, very fast.* And while it is true that today the chance of an American woman's being infected is still very small, this is not likely to be true tomorrow. Our information about women and AIDS in Africa, where it is widespread among men and women, albeit not precise, is alarming. It is therefore difficult to predict as the mushrooming cloud of this plague darkens the land how far it will reach and whether we are going to share the tragic fate of our African sisters.

3. Infected Women Give Birth to Babies with Aids.

One of my most personally compelling reasons for trying to reach out to women is that too few know that once infected, you carry the AIDS virus in your bloodstream, presumably *for life*. This means that once you become infected, you not only stand a good chance of coming down with AIDS, but if you become pregnant, your baby is at great risk of catching the virus from you during the pregnancy, and probably 50 percent of your future babies are going to be born with AIDS and die during early childhood.† Infants have also contracted AIDS through their infected mother's milk. So if you think that there is even a remote possibility that you have been exposed, please take an AIDS test to make sure you are not a carrier before you decide to get pregnant or to nurse your baby.

---

* Here is a simplified illustration of a *geometric increase*, where growth is by multiplication and is rapid, as opposed to an arithmetic increase, where growth is by addition, and is slow.

If you take one penny and double it you get two pennies, which is still very little, but if you continue doubling, you get 4, then 8, 16, 32, 64, $1.24, $2.48, $4.96, $9.92, $19.94 — and before you know it you are doubling millions of dollars!

In terms of women and AIDS, we are still talking about pennies. But we might be seeing millions of AIDS cases if we do not prevent the spread.

† Scientific References, Group II: AIDS in Children and Transmission of HIV from Infected Mothers to Their Babies During Pregnancy.

The tragedy of infant infection has up to now rarely been mentioned in public AIDS education programs or on AIDS hotlines, and this deeply troubling aspect of AIDS certainly has not been sufficiently stressed in public health prevention programs. Perhaps the AIDS babies issue has been neglected because educational campaigns have been mainly targeting the high-risk male homosexuals and drug users. I also believe that perhaps the special hazards of the transmission of AIDS from mother to fetus, and AIDS in newborns, have not been addressed for political reasons.

Religious groups who are against contraception and abortion might not be eager to raise this touchy issue because many physicians are now recommending abortions for seropositive* women, and most health authorities are advising contraception to prevent future pregnancies.

I think that perhaps one reason gay activists also would rather not talk about babies born with AIDS is because they do not want the public's attention diverted away from the problems facing them in terms of their job security and potential insurance problems. The reasons why those two interest groups are playing down issues related to women's health and to birth are understandable expressions of their own special concerns.

But why the American Civil Liberties Union, a privately funded agency which mounts legal actions on behalf of certain constitutional issues, has made the prevention of potential civil liberties abuses such an overwhelming priority is beyond my comprehension. †

A policy statement issued by the ACLU on Communi-

---

* You will often see the word *seropositive* in this book, which essentially means that the person is infected with AIDS. More specifically the term *seropositive* means the person's blood, actually the liquid part of the blood known as "serum," contains antibodies to the AIDS virus. This indicates that the virus has invaded his or her body. Seropositive individuals are infectious to their babies and to others because their organs and body fluids are full of AIDS virus. In the United States at this time the great majority of seropositive persons (100 to 1) are asymptomatic "carriers" of the AIDS virus and have no outward signs or symptoms of the disease.

† See Appendix A.

cable Diseases and AIDS in 1986 acknowledged that "Government actions designed to control communicable diseases raise serious civil liberties concerns. There is a tension between public health requirements and civil liberties standards." The document describes the ACLU's policies on AIDS antibody testing and on warning the sexual partners of persons with HIV infection as follows, "Compulsory sexual contact tracing with respect to AIDS raises grave civil liberties concerns because the major identifiable groups that are most at risk are deeply discriminated against. In this context, the possibility that the government may acquire the authority to collect the names of people in such groups is ominous.*

I would think that the rights of women to be informed that they are in danger of being infected with a fatal disease should take precedence over potential breaches of an HIV carrier's right to privacy. I consider discrimination terrible, but far less ominous than the enormous tragedy of babies being born with AIDS, or of young women's loss of the ability to bear healthy children.

The unthinkable horror that more and more children are being subjected to the ultimate abuse of being born to die of AIDS, simply because their mothers had received insufficient or misleading information on safe sex, or because AIDS testing was not available, is to me the most shocking example of how criminally negligent our public health policies have been in relation to women. It is crucial that women and young teenagers, two groups who possibly face the greatest imminent risk, wake up to these facts and demand some changes!

4. No One Will Protect You Except Yourself.

The main reason I am addressing this book to women is that it is ultimately every woman's own responsibility to protect herself and her yet unborn babies.

---

* ACLU National Policy on Communicable Diseases and AIDS, American Civil Liberties Union Foundation, New York, 1986.

It is your life and your body.

You cannot expect your man to protect you. He may not know how.

Your doctor cannot be counted on to protect you. Primary care physicians are just beginning to learn about AIDS, and in many communities your doctor's hands have been tied by politics. Did you know that in some American communities it is actually against the medical society's and/ or the health department's policies for a doctor to inform anyone except the patient that his AIDS test indicates he is infected, unless the patient gives his consent? For example, in New York City, which has the highest rate of HIV infection in the country, the health department even advises physicians not to tell *the wife of an AIDS carrier* that her husband is infected and that she is in mortal danger, if her infected husband does not give his consent! All in the interests of protecting the HIV carrier's "right to privacy."

I believe that the confidentiality of a patient's communications with his physician must be respected. But a doctor's obligation to protect clearly identified potential victims, in this case wife and offspring, should come first.

The law will certainly not protect you. And politicians can't be expected to change the law unless people demand a change.

Women must learn to take care of themselves in all areas of their lives, but this is particularly difficult when it comes to sex. Because we have been trained to be "good girls" from infancy on, it is hard for many well-brought-up women to assert themselves in this sensitive, vulnerable matter of sexuality. And the irony and tragedy is that the sweetest, the nicest, the gentlest, the most loving, the most sensitive young women, the women who do not wish to hurt a man's feelings by questioning his integrity, or his masculinity, who find it easier to *give* than to *take,* who hate to ask for anything that is not freely volunteered— these are the women who are the most likely victims of this plague.

2

The Politics of AIDS: Women and Children Last

Everyone knows by now that AIDS is a fatal disease. Unless we find the cure soon, which is highly unlikely, every person who now has AIDS is expected to die. Since the disease was unknown before 1978, no one can tell as yet if anyone is immune or resistant or just how many persons infected with the virus will eventually succumb. We already know that a large proportion of carriers * will ultimately fall victim to the disease, because between 25 percent to 50 percent of those who have been infected have developed AIDS within seven years from the time the virus entered the body. Every year more are expected to become ill and then die. To add to the tragedy, AIDS-related illnesses and deaths are often cruelly painful.

* A *carrier* is a person who is infected with the AIDS virus and is therefore infectious to others, but who has no outward signs or symptoms of AIDS. You may also see *"healthy"* carriers referred to by the medical term "asymptomatic," which means "without visible symptoms."

IT IS NOT TOO LATE TO PROTECT WOMEN, BUT IT'S CLOSE

The AIDS epidemic is now moving to its seventh documented year in the United States.

The disease was first reported in this country in 1981 in a few male homosexuals, although in retrospect, cases may have been appearing as early as 1978. It then spread to intravenous drug users. Male homosexuals and drug users are now very heavily infected, and they make up 90 percent of all the AIDS cases reported to date. The remaining 10 percent is mostly made up of recipients of contaminated blood or blood products (this includes hemophiliacs, who depend on blood products for their survival), and children of infected mothers.

As of this year a total of 2207 cases of AIDS in women had been reported to the CDC. Sixty-three percent have already died, and the heterosexual transmission rate is increasing rapidly (see Table 1). Dr. Anthony Fauci, the director of the National Institute of Allergy and Infectious Diseases, commenting on the rapidly rising rate of heterosexual transmission, estimated that "we expect 10 percent of U.S. AIDS cases to be heterosexually transmitted by 1991."*

The disease has spread alarmingly. As of the end of 1986, 28,098 cases of AIDS had been reported in the United States. But only two months later the number had jumped to 31,036. The Centers for Disease Control estimates that two million Americans are now infected with the AIDS virus.

In June 1986 the U.S. Public Health Service held a conference on AIDS in Berkeley Springs, West Virginia, bringing together top AIDS experts, epidemiologists, specialists in infectious diseases, virologists, pathologists, and public

* Scientific References, Group I: The Epidemiology of AIDS.

Figure 1 *Distribution of U.S. Adult AIDS Patients*

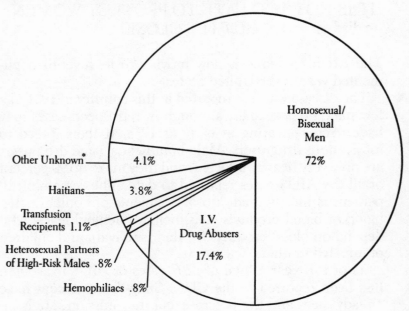

Homosexual/
Bisexual
Men

72%

Other Unknown* — 4.1%

Haitians — 3.8%

Transfusion
Recipients 1.1%

I.V.
Drug Abusers

Heterosexual Partners
of High-Risk Males .8%

17.4%

Hemophiliacs .8%

*Included in this category are patients who could not be placed in a known risk group or who died before an accurate history could be taken.

Source: *Morbidity & Mortality Weekly Report*, Centers for Disease Control, U.S. Dept. of Health and Human Services 33(24): June 22, 1984.

health officials. According to Dr. P. J. Imperato, who summarized the conference in a recent issue of the *N.Y. State Journal of Medicine*, "Among the troubling predictions that came from that meeting was that by 1991, only four short years from now, there will be more than a quarter million (250,000) cases of AIDS in the United States."* Many of the new cases are expected to occur in drug-free heterosexual men and women.

Dr. Imperato went on to report: "It was also predicted that in the same short period of time at least 54,000 more

* Dr. Pascal James Imperato is the chairman of the Department of Preventive Medicine at the S.U.N.Y. Health Science Center, Brooklyn, N.Y. The quotation comes from his editorial remarks in the May edition of the *New York State Journal of Medicine*, which was devoted to the AIDS epidemic.

people will have died of AIDS in the United States, ironi-
cally this is approximately the same number of Americans
who died during the last fifteen years of the Vietnam War."
Up to now, the disease has struck down mostly young people.

Many experts think that current estimates of the spread
of the disease are actually much too low because they are
based on faulty numbers. There are no federal laws requir-
ing doctors and hospitals to report AIDS carriers, and in
many cases physicians — in order to protect the families
and the reputations of the victims — are not listing the
disease as a cause of death.

It has been estimated that for every case of AIDS there

Figure 2 *Patients with AIDS and Carriers*

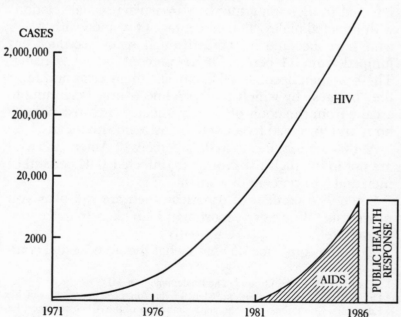

NOTE: This graph shows the increase in AIDS infection in the United States between
1971 and 1986, and also estimates the relationship, 1 to 100, of patients with AIDS to
"healthy" AIDS carriers.

Source: Robert R. Redfield, M.D., and Donald S. Burke, M.D., "Shadow on the Land:
The Epidemiology of HIV Infection," *American Journal of Immunology*, 1987.

are now *one hundred* healthy carriers who are capable of transmitting the disease through sex, blood, or pregnancy, presumably for the rest of their lives.* It is not known just how many infected men do not realize they are carriers, but I would guess there are many.† This lack of awareness is terrible for women, for how can you expect a man to protect you if he does not know that he is infectious?

The disease is currently still largely confined to two relatively small groups of high-risk males: homosexuals who have given AIDS to each other through sexual contact so that in some communities the majority are infected, and I.V. drug users, who are contaminating each other on a continuous basis by sharing their needles. Until this year heterosexual transmission of AIDS virus to women was rare, but no longer. Unfortunately women are becoming infected in increasing numbers by having sexual relations with infected males. The percentage of women with AIDS who have become infected through *sexual contact* has jumped from 14 percent to 26 percent — and is rising. These women become AIDS carriers themselves and form the "bridges" by which the epidemic is now beginning to escape from the pools of heavily infected high-risk populations and to spread to general mainstream Americans.‡

At this writing, less than 0.03 percent of Americans who are not in the high-risk groups are infected: 0.04 percent of men and 0.01 percent of women.

Since 99.6 percent of American men are still okay you might ask, "Why worry, most men I am likely to make love to are safe!"

Don't be complacent! That's what the homosexual com-

* Scientific References, Group I, The Epidemiology of AIDS.
† Dr. Theresa Crenshaw, past president of the American Association of Sex Educators, Counselors, and Therapists, and chair of the AIDS task force, has stated that 90% of HIV carriers are not aware of their AIDS status.
‡ Until 1986, more than one-half of American women with AIDS were infected by drug abuse. In 1986, the cases contracted by heterosexual transmission began to increase faster than those due to infection from contaminated needles. At this writing, sex with an infected man holds the most danger for women. Scientific References, Group I: The Epidemiology of AIDS.

munity thought six years ago, and now only 30 percent are free of the AIDS virus in some communities; of the 70 percent who are infected, as many as half are expected to die!*

The epidemic is spreading very rapidly.

We have every reason to believe Dr. Imperato's gloomy statement that "it is clear that 1987 represents the year in the AIDS epidemic where heterosexual transmission becomes an important concern."

Many experts believe that adolescents and teenagers are especially vulnerable. As of 1987 only a few hundred teenagers have been identified as having AIDS by the Centers for Disease Control, but there are alarming signs that high schools, especially those in inner cities, may soon become disaster areas for the heterosexual transmission of AIDS. Some leading experts, including Dr. Karen Hein, a professor of Pediatrics at the Albert Einstein College of Medicine, believe that a large number of young infected I.V. drug users and adolescent males who have had sex with infected homosexual men are just beginning to become sexually active. Few of these young carriers, or the girls in their classes, have the slightest idea that they have been infected, and they are spreading AIDS through heterosexual contact within their peer groups.

HOW DO WE STOP IT?

You might hear that the whole blame lies with the government for not spending enough money on AIDS research, a view expressed by Congressman Ted Weiss from New York.† It is true that one can never spend too much for saving lives. But in fact, thanks largely to the foresight and tremendous effort on the part of the homosexual commu-

* Scientific References, Group I, The Epidemiology of AIDS.
† AIDS: *Facts and Issues*, Victor Gong, M.D., and Norman Rudnick, Editors. Rutgers University Press, 1986.

nity to fight AIDS, there has been an unprecedented international effort to combat this killer disease, and astounding advances have been made in a very short time. In just five years of research, scientists have already discovered the *cause* of AIDS (the AIDS virus, also known as HIV, the Human Immunodeficiency Virus [formerly called HTLV-III/LAV]); its route of *transmission* (mainly through sex, blood, and pregnancy); and have developed excellent *tests* that can detect persons who are *carriers* with great accuracy.

This is extremely rapid progress when we consider that we still have no cure for most cancers after eighty years of intensive research, and that it took twenty-five years or so to develop a vaccine for polio! But there is still no AIDS cure or vaccine in sight — nor is there likely to be for a long time, because the disease is caused by a retrovirus (explained later on). This type of virus is so complex (much more complex for example than the polio virus) that it is technically extremely difficult to make vaccines or find cures.

Until we have a remedy we must rely on *prevention*. That is not as bad as it sounds. Prevention can be extremely effective. For example, public health education campaigns, which raised America's consciousness about the dangers of a fatty diet and high blood pressure, have reduced the incidence of heart attack and stroke by 60 percent in the last ten years!

THE POLITICS OF AIDS

Scientists and epidemiologists know how to control the spread of infectious diseases like AIDS. There is every reason to believe that they could succeed if it were politically feasible to deal with AIDS as with other sexually transmitted diseases.

Public health experts and organizations, including the U.S. Public Health Service's Centers for Disease Control and the World Health Organization, have recommended a comprehensive program of prevention that includes public education, the wide use of AIDS testing, the avoidance of casual sex with high-risk or infected persons, and risk-reducing procedures such as safe sexual practices and the use of condoms.

More specifically, public health experts have recommended educational programs that tell the truth about AIDS. But no single educational program can effectively protect everyone. Each new risk group has different needs and problems and each needs an individual education program that fits its particular circumstances. Right now we have sensible and effective programs for high-risk males who make up 93 percent of AIDS cases. But women and adolescents, who are about to be hit by this epidemic, need a public health program with a totally different approach, and this is *not* being done.

The great majority of public health experts recommend that AIDS testing be made widely available so that carriers can be identified, and counseled so that they understand that they are infectious to others. *All feel the tests results should be kept confidential.* But there is no unanimity about *who* should be tested, and whether testing should be *anonymous.** Some infectious disease specialists think that only vulnerable groups at risk of becoming infected — such as women who are pregnant, blood donors and semen donors, and partners of high-risk men — should be tested. (To which I would urgently add adolescents in the high schools and junior high schools, especially in high-risk areas.) Some doctors have recommended compulsory testing of groups that present special public health hazards, including immigrants (especially those from highly infected

* *Anonymous* testing means that one can take the AIDS antibody tests without having to give one's name. This can be done at *alternate testing sites*, which are now available in some communities. In contrast, you have to identify yourself if you are tested confidentially, but the records are not available to any unauthorized person or organization. For information on alternate testing sites or confidential testing, call your local health department or medical society.

places such as Haiti or Central Africa), couples applying for a marriage license (who are currently required to be tested for syphilis in some states), and patients who are being admitted to hospitals, for surgical procedures where infected blood is a possible danger to healthcare workers. Many public health officials have recommended that doctors should be required by law to report individuals who are infected with the AIDS virus because they feel that is the only way that the disease can be tracked. Others disagree because of the fear of discrimination against gays and drug addicts. Many have also stated that tracing and informing *contacts* would be helpful. This standard public health procedure for controlling infectious diseases involves finding persons (the "contacts") who may have been infected and are therefore unknowingly infecting others.

Contact tracing has been successful in limiting the spread of many contagious diseases before cures and vaccines were available. Many years ago the health department traced a number of persons who became ill with typhoid fever to a restaurant. There they found that a food handler who was not ill herself, but was a "carrier" of the typhoid baccillus, had been spreading the infection to patrons of the restaurant. At the time we did not yet have a remedy for typhoid, so "Typhoid Mary," as she came to be nicknamed, was asked to find another line of work.

It is currently the consensus of scientists that AIDS is not transmitted through food or casual contact, only through the exchange of body fluids. This exchange occurs mainly by way of sex, blood, and pregnancy, so it makes no sense to quarantine AIDS patients or to restrict their employment. But many leading authorities believe that tracing of contacts could save many lives. Potentially infected persons, most of whom *do not know* they were exposed, could also be tested and, if found to be infected, counseled not to donate blood or sperm, and to protect their sexual partners.

Although today 27 percent of AIDS carriers are thought to be heterosexually active, bisexuals and I.V. drug users, so that AIDS is no longer an exclusively "gay disease," the fact that AIDS started in the homosexual community in this country and that male gays are still the most heavily infected group in America, has had profound political consequences on the AIDS situation.

The intense and successful effort on the part of the homosexual community early on to raise the world's consciousness about the need for research and funding for AIDS has yielded all of us enormous benefits. We now have the tests and the knowledge we need to control the disease. But the problems created by the gay community's special vulnerability to and concern about potential discrimination and civil rights abuses, are obstructing the proper use of this hard-won technology. These concerns are now seriously interfering with protecting women and adolescents from the oncoming epidemic. Unfortunately, and through no one's fault, the policies that are good for the health and the civil liberties of homosexual males, are now in some respects in direct conflict with what is in the best interests of women and children.

The various organizations and groups who are struggling with each other on opposing sides of the AIDS testing and condoms questions are by and large well-intentioned people with nothing personal to gain, who believe they are doing the right thing. *But the struggle itself is destructive.* The struggle is paralyzing public health efforts and causing the dissemination of misinformation and disinformation which is terribly dangerous for women.

A brief look at the history of AIDS in this country will explain how and why this is happening.

When it became apparent that this disease had struck the homosexual community five or six years ago, there was great and understandable concern that the AIDS epidemic would result in a backlash against homosexuals. Gay activists were particularly afraid of AIDS testing, fearing that mandatory reporting of AIDS carriers, who were predominantly homosexuals, could be misused and could lead to discrimination against infected individuals.

To protect their rights and their lifestyles and their sexual freedom, they enlisted the help of civil rights organizations* and mounted an intense and well-organized, well-funded campaign against AIDS testing and mandatory reporting of carriers. Some responsible and enlightened gay activist groups, as for example those in San Francisco and London, have recognized the value of testing to themselves and to others; they have made extensive use of the AIDS test technology, but have wisely insisted that the confidentiality of the records should be strictly protected. These organizations have properly pressed for laws to protect the civil rights of carriers, which makes a great deal of sense to me.

But other organizations, most especially the ACLU and the LAMBDA Legal Defense (a gay rights legal organization), are working against AIDS testing, tracing of contacts, and/or reporting of AIDS carriers to health authorities,† which are regarded by many public health experts as essential for control of the epidemic.‡ The concern for HIV carriers' rights to privacy seems to be overwhelming to these groups. Groups with these same political positions, for example, in New York City, had been promoting advertising campaigns and educational material that by implication exaggerate the degree of safety provided by condoms.§

But it has been known all along that condoms only *reduce the risk* of sexual exposure but *do not eliminate* it. While risk-reduction policies make sense for protecting high-risk homosexual males, many of whose potential partners are already infected, it is wrong and dangerous to urge women and adolescents to place their futures in condoms to reduce the risks of sexual exposure. Since the great majority of heterosexual men who do not shoot drugs

* *ACLU National Policy on Communicable Diseases and AIDS*, American Civil Liberties Union Foundation, New York, 1986.
† See Appendix B.
‡Scientific References Group IV: The AIDS Tests, Counseling, and Prevention.
§ See Appendix C.

are healthy, it is far easier and much safer for women to simply *avoid sexual exposure to high-risk males* with really safe "dry sex" and AIDS testing (as will be explained in Chapter 4).

On the other side of the struggle are some lawmakers and certain religious leaders who are understandably deeply concerned about the potential moral dangers which they see as inherent in public sex education campaigns. They fear that the public sanctioning of condoms, with the implicit acceptance of sex outside of marriage and of homosexuality, threatens to erode the religious and ethical values to which they are committed. They fear the moral fiber of the entire nation is at stake and they want to protect the traditional values of marriage, family, and monogamy by confining children's sex education to the home and the church or synagogue. On these grounds, the Roman Catholic Church, the Orthodox Jewish rabbinate, and a number of other conservative religious and political organizations are opposed to condom advertisements in the media. These groups want to limit educational and counseling programs to emphasizing the avoidance of promiscuous sex, and to promoting monogamy and chastity. Some go so far as to oppose any form of sex education outside the home, and object to the very mention of sex in the schools or in the media. They do not seem to understand that explicit public education programs are crucial to the success of public health efforts to control AIDS.

Unfortunately a few bigots seem to be trying to use the AIDS crisis as an opportunity to vent their antihomosexual bias. Some of these individuals have made outrageous and irrational proposals, such as mandatory quarantine or imprisonment of all homosexuals regardless of their AIDS status. But they represent a *tiny, crazy minority*. There are also a few radical groups on the other side who, despite the clear need for available AIDS testing, do not seem to appreciate how many lives could be lost in their strenuous opposition to even voluntary testing. Although testing is considered essential by many experts for preventing the spread of AIDS to the general population, certain organizations are doing their best to discourage even voluntary testing. For example, a pamphlet entitled "Medical Answers About AIDS," by L. Mass, M.D., which was distributed by the Gay Men's Health Crisis (GMHC, Inc.) in 1987 states about the AIDS antibody test: ". . . It is not a test for AIDS. It is a test to determine if an individual has been exposed to AIDS. . . . Many people who feel that they are at risk for AIDS will want to be immediately tested. They should be strongly urged not to seek the test at this time."

With the exceptions of a few such extremists, however, the majority of people who hold opposing views about AIDS are well-meaning individuals who have been blinded by their desires to do what they consider right. They are essentially people of integrity who are simply deeply committed to defending their value systems, which they feel are being threatened.

Moreover, it is difficult even for experts to keep up with all the new information that is constantly pouring in. Politicians and activist groups and legal groups are not scientists and most of them are not well informed about the actual scientific and medical facts regarding the disease, and they don't seem to understand that their opposition to testing and their exaggeration of the safety of condoms could have deadly consequences, or that countless lives could be lost if public sex education were to be prohibited altogether. The opposing factions are putting their own agendas ahead of concern for the safety of women and children, who may well be decimated by the oncoming epidemic.

But it really makes no practical difference whether the motives of the various interest groups are evil or pure. The only thing that matters is that the *result* of their fighting is destructive to you, and the only thing which is really important is that *you learn to protect yourself.*

As I have sometimes said to patients in an effort to motivate them to put their energy into taking care of themselves, instead of wasting time on self-pity or anger at others: "If a bird soils your head, it doesn't matter if it was aiming at you or just had to relieve itself. What matters is that you clean yourself up and make sure no one fouls you up again!"

I am dwelling on how this country's shameful neglect of women and children regarding AIDS came about because I believe that the greater your understanding, the easier it will be for you to commit yourself to doing something about it.

We live in a democracy and it is only natural that politicians mostly worry first and foremost about winning the next election so that they can keep their jobs. Therefore many of our elected leaders are waiting to see which way the public will vote before they take a definite position or any action on AIDS.

With this in mind, the groups with different special interests, the thoughtful and the crazies, the gay extremists and the fundamental Judeo-Christian religious groups, the ultraconservatives and the ultraliberals, the civil rights activists and the Moral Majority, are all trying to sway public opinion with emotional and often inaccurate and misleading campaigns.

Meanwhile everything is at a standstill and the public health measures and educational programs have not been changed to accommodate *women's* needs. In their present form, AIDS prevention programs and AIDS-related health legislation are at best inadequate and in fact actually *destructive* to women and children and, ultimately of course, to heterosexual men as well.

One of the aspects of the struggle between the antitest and the anticondom factions that is most dangerous for women is that it has produced a great deal of misinformation and confusion about what is safe and what is not safe.

For example, on Sunday, May 17, 1987, the highly respected *New York Times* carried an editorial that objected to AIDS tests on the erroneous grounds that there are too many "false positives,"* that is, too many people will get a positive reading on their initial screening test, even though they are not infected with the AIDS virus. The editorial expressed concern that this will cause emotional trauma to people who are wrongly told that they have AIDS.

On May 5, 1987, *The New York Times* published a letter by Mark Barnes, an Associate in Law at Columbia University, entitled "AIDS Test Is, Unfortunately, Still Ambiguous," which exaggerated the ambiguity of the tests even further. Mr. Barnes wrote that "estimates on the number of false positives . . . range from a majority . . . to as high as 90% on all samples testing positive on the ELISA test."†

What total nonsense! In a subsequent letter to *The New York Times*, Dr. Michael Marmor, in the Department of Infectious Diseases at New York University, corrected this and explained that in fact *two* tests are used in combination to make the diagnosis of HIV infection: a *screening test* (ELISA), which is *always* followed in case of a positive result by a second screening test to make sure that the laboratory did not make a mistake, and then, if still positive, an *extremely accurate confirming test* (Western blot) is performed. Only then is a person told that he or she is infected.‡ The accuracy of this combination of tests is over 99 percent, which is much higher than that of many of the tests used to detect a number of cancers and other diseases.§ Nevertheless, any large-scale screening will produce a *tiny* number of false positives, and no one wants to cause even a single person unnecessary emotional pain. But in view of the many deaths and tragedies that could be prevented by making AIDS testing widely available, the benefits far outweigh the risks. I share Dr. Marmor's concern that this kind of discouragement of AIDS testing can have potentially "lethal consequences."

And even more upsetting to me as a physician are the

---

* See appendixes E, A, F, and G.
† Letter to *The New York Times*, May 5, 1987.
‡ See Appendix G.
§ Scientific References, Group IV: The AIDS Tests, Counseling, and Prevention.

York City Health Department up until May 1987! These TV spots left the distinct impression that as long as you wear a condom you can safely have sex. Condoms do *reduce* the risk of exposure, although no one knows by how much. However, every public health doctor is perfectly aware that the level of protection is nowhere close to 100 percent!

It seems clear to me that we could save the lives of significant numbers of women, babies, and adolescents by pointing out the fact that it is much safer for these groups to *eliminate* the risk of infection by avoiding sexual exposure to high-risk males.

You have a right to accurate information, and, it is incumbent on our society to see to it that you know the whole truth, because you and your offspring can survive only if you are well informed.

WHY OUR PREVENTION POLICIES ARE NOT GOOD FOR WOMEN AND CHILDREN

Public AIDS prevention policies in the U.S. were originally designed for controlling the AIDS epidemic that was spreading like wildfire in the male homosexual community. These policies were naturally tailored to fit the unique sexual behavior patterns and also the special vulnerability to discrimination of male homosexuals.

But, although heterosexual women are at increasingly greater risk, this country is still using essentially the same risk-reducing approach that was appropriate and made sense for controlling the disease among male gays. But no one seems to be taking into consideration the striking and significant differences in the sexual behavior patterns of women and adolescents, or the potential risks of the entire population's exposure to the AIDS virus, or the civil rights of heterosexuals, which are in some respects in conflict with gay rights.

It is incredible that almost no one, not even women themselves, seems to be acknowledging that AIDS *risk-*

reduction programs, which have had and still have an important place for AIDS prevention among male gays, are wrong for women, for whom the only policy that makes sense is the *elimination* of risks, by avoiding sex with infected males!* Moreover there has been enormous resistance to passing new laws that would facilitate the identification of male AIDS carriers, who clearly present the greatest danger for women today. It seems impossible to get any support for prevention programs that meet the special needs of women and their as yet unborn babies, and this is most urgent for young adolescent girls, who may soon be ravaged by the oncoming epidemic.

INFECTED PARTNERS

Let's look at some of the differences between low-risk women and high-risk males.

It has been estimated that from 50 to 70 percent of male homosexuals and bisexuals in the large gay communities in San Francisco and New York City are currently infected with the AIDS virus. † It follows that at least half of the potential homosexual partners of gay men are already infected, and unless a gay man is in a long-term monogamous relationship, he will either have to give up sex or try to *reduce* the risk.

A main difference between women and gay males, one that underlies the thrust of programs to prevent the spread of this sexually transmitted disease, is that male homosexuals tend as a group to have many, many more partners than heterosexual (or homosexual) women, and they have sex with strangers far more frequently.

---

* The front page of a recent (1987) edition of *EIDOS*, a newspaper for the "Erotic Entertainment of Women," featured the headline "15,000 Condoms" with a photograph of young men and women marching on behalf of "Safe Sex" with the Bill Baird AIDS Awareness Fund. The organization advocates promoting condoms, and on the second page of the paper was the announcement that "15,000 Ramses condoms . . . will be distributed free at the Arlington Street Church along the march. . . ."

† Scientific References, Group I: The Epidemiology of AIDS.

I.V. drug using males are rapidly reaching the same saturation point of infection in inner-city ghettos, especially in the New York metropolitan area. It has been estimated that there are 500,000 narcotics addicts in the United States, that in some areas up to 60 percent may be infected, and that the prevalence is directly related to their distance from New York City. It may be speculated that I.V. drug using men are more sexually active and more promiscuous than women of the same social class, but this has not been established.*

Although many male gays are in monogamous relationships, especially those who are older, and especially today, clinical experience indicates that the freedom to have sex with multiple partners is very important to many.

This is expresseed in Dennis Altman's highly acclaimed book, *AIDS in the Mind of America* (Anchor Books, 1987), "To fundamentally alter sexual behavior (to try to become monogamous) is considerably more far reaching than giving up smoking or drinking, at least for some people. For gay men a certain sexual lifestyle is inextricably intertwined with being gay." Altman goes on to quote David Black (*The Plague Years*, Simon and Schuster, 1987), "For gay men sex, that most powerful implement of attachment and arousal, is also an agent of communion, replacing an often hostile family and even shaping politics. It represents an ecstatic break with years of glances and guises, the furtive past we left behind."

It is quite common for a male homosexual to have more than a thousand partners during his life.† And gay men tend to have sexual encounters with partners they do not know far more frequently than heterosexual men and women do (see Table 3).

Current public health programs and the laws that sup-

---

* Scientific References, Group I, The Epidemiology of AIDS.
† These figures come from Bell and Weinberg's *Homosexualities*, a superb demographic study of the sexual behaviors of more than 1500 homosexual men and women in San Francisco. The survey, which was sponsored by the Kinsey Institute, was published in 1978, just when the AIDS epidemic was silently beginning to invade the gay community.

Table 3 *Homosexual Behavior Patterns**

A. NUMBERS OF SEXUAL PARTNERS

Number of Homosexual Partners Ever	WHH (N=574)	BHM (N=111)	WHF (N=227)	BHF (N=64)	PILOT STUDY (N=458)
0: 1	0%	0%	3%	5%	
1: 2	0	0	9	5	
2: 3–4	1	2	15	14	1%
3: 5–9	2	4	31	30	3
4: 10–14	3	5	16	9	4
5: 15–24	3	6	10	16	5
6: 25–49	8	6	8	11	8
7: 50–99	9	18	5	8	12
8: 100–249	15	15	1	2	20
9: 250–499	17	11	1	2	13
10: 500–999	15	14	0	0	14
11: 1000 or more	28	19	0	0	20

WHM = White homosexual men
BHM = Black homosexual men
WHF = White homosexual females
BHF = Black homosexual females

B. CASUAL SEXUAL PARTNERS

Proportion of Partners Who Were Strangers	(N=574)	(N=111)	(N=225)	(N=64)	(N=458)
0: None	1%	5%	62%	56%	6%
1–3: Half or less	20	43	32	38	26
4–6: More than half	79	51	6	6	68

Proportion of Partners with Whom R† Had Sex Only Once	(N=572)	(N=111)	(N=225)	(N=64)	(N=458)
0: None	1%	4%	38%	41%	3%
1–3: Half or less	29	59	51	55	40
4–6: More than half	70	38	12	5	57

Source: *Homosexualities*, by A. P. Bell and M. S. Weinberg, N.Y., Simon and Schuster, 1978.

*Note that 28% of white homosexual males reported having had sex with more than 1,000 different sexual partners, while 79% admitted that more than one-half of their partners were strangers.
†R refers to "Respondent" (the person who answered the researcher's questions).

port them were designed with these circumstances in mind, as well as with appropriate concern for protecting the homosexual community from a potential antigay backlash and from civil rights infringements. And those policies are right for gays at risk.

Since in some homosexual communities the majority of the partners available to those homosexual men who are still uninfected are AIDS carriers, the advice given by many AIDS hotlines and educational campaigns is that the best way to reduce risk to sexually active gay men who are not infected is to assume that everyone has been exposed and therefore to practice "safe sex." Safe sex for gay men is defined as using condoms and avoiding "high-risk" sexual behavior (presumably unprotected anal sex with strangers in "high-risk" locales, such as gay bars and bathhouses). The formation of "Jack Off Clubs" is also recommended. *

This advice makes a great deal of sense for reducing the risks entailed in homosexual exposure for men who wish to continue to have multiple partners. And, while I do not agree from the point of view of good public health practices, and most especially because discouraging testing may have lethal effects for women and adolescents, I can understand the "THE TEST CAN BE ALMOST AS DEVASTATING AS THE DISEASE"† campaigns as an

---

* The Institute for the Advanced Study of Human Sexuality recommends a videotape called "How to Have a J.O. (Jack Off) Party" (*Safe Sex in the Age of AIDS*, Institute for the Advanced Study of Human Sexuality, 1986). Dennis Altman, in his book *AIDS in the Mind of America* (Anchor Books, 1987), also describes J.O. clubs in which members join to watch each other masturbate and come to orgasm. This is certainly safe from the standpoint of AIDS.

† The GMHC, Inc. (Gay Men's Health Crisis) distributed a leaflet with that title in 1985. The leaflet has a photograph of the nude torso of a handsome male and contains the warning that "what it [the AIDS antibody test] can do is frightening. Imagine if your health insurance company found out that your test came back positive, they might cancel your policy. Even your job and home may be at risk. Names might be reported to the government and find their way onto a master list. . . . Our advice is to stay away from the test. It's bad news." (In fact, insurance companies cannot cancel policies for conditions that occur after a policy has been taken out.)

expression of the gay community's concern about the potential for civil rights infringements.

But the focus of this book is women, and the circumstances for women are completely different. We need a different approach. It is wrong for the AIDS hotlines to give our young women the same advice they give to high-risk men and to obfuscate the failure rates of condoms. And I think it is especially wrong that when a woman who is worried about being exposed to AIDS, and worried about infecting her future partners and offspring, calls the New York City Health Department AIDS Hotline for advice, she is given misleading information. There is something very wrong when a woman caller is *repeatedly* told that her future babies are not in danger, that she has nothing to worry about, and that she doesn't need to be tested "if your partner wore a condom." *

Women do not mind monogamy and sexual exclusivity as much as gay men do; in fact, many prefer sex in a committed relationship. Women as a group have always been more interested in the *quality* of sex rather than *quantity* provided by different partners. There are, of course, some women who like to have multiple sexual encounters with strangers. However, the great majority of heterosexual as well as homosexual women have a much more modest number of sexual partners than gay men. Women are also more likely to know their partners better because "one-night stands," and "scoring," are far less popular with women.

But the most important difference between low-risk females and high-risk males, based on U.S. blood bank studies, is that only a tiny proportion of women's potential partners, † actually less than four in ten thousand (0.04 percent), are infected at this time even in the high-risk areas like New York, Washington D.C. and San Francisco, and even less than that in low-risk areas.

* See Appendix C.
† If they are not bisexuals, I.V. drug users, or hemophiliacs.

Figure 3 *AIDS Cases by State in the United States to October 21, 1985*

(N = 14,288)

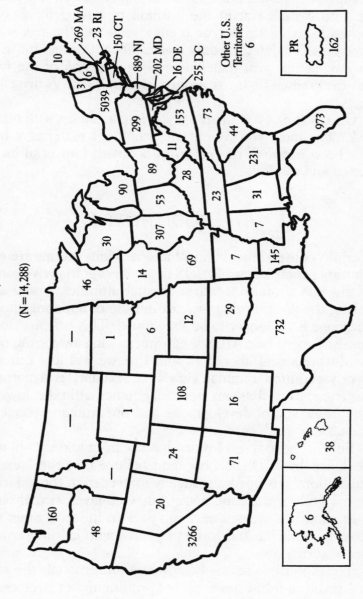

269 MA
23 RI
150 CT
889 NJ
202 MD
16 DE
255 DC

Other U.S.
Territories
6

PR
162

10
3 6
5039
299
153
73
44
973
231
11
89
28
23
31
90
53
7
30
307
7
145
46
14
69
7
1
6
12
29
732
—
1
108
16
—
1
24
71
—
20
3266
160
48

38

6

Source: Centers for Disease Control, Center for Infectious Diseases AIDS Branch

47

Please remember, the great majority of your potential sexual partners are not infected or infectious! At this point in time we are not in the position of having to choose between giving up sex or merely reducing the risk with condoms. To date, the only real significant danger for us is in having sex with males who belong to one of the two relatively small high-risk groups: bisexuals or I.V. drug addicts.

Clearly the best strategy for you is to avoid sex with high-risk men, and if you are not sure whether a man has or has not been exposed, do not go to bed with him until he is tested and cleared!

THE GOOD NEWS

Certain conservative political and religious groups are exploiting people's fear of AIDS in an attempt to revive some of the old moralism and antisexual attitudes. Some are taking the position that any sex outside of a monogamous marriage is no longer to be sanctioned. This has produced some concern that AIDS is causing a swing away from our hard-won sexual liberation, and that we will lose our recently acquired rational view that sexuality is a natural function, as well as our new enlightened attitudes toward children's sexual development and our humane concern for sexual health care.

But the "sexual revolution" has not been and should not be killed by AIDS. I hope and believe that the "sexual revolution" has freed our society forever from the old irrational guilt and shame about our God-given sexual feelings. And that we will never go back to the days when we used to ostracize and torment people who led unconventional sexual lives.

To responsible sexual health care professionals the sexual revolution has never meant promiscuity or irresponsible sexual behavior. It is true that AIDS has put an end to casual sex with strangers, but I don't consider this a loss.

In fact to me, the one silver lining in the dreadful AIDS cloud is that people will have to get to know each other better and develop an intimate, trusting, and caring relationship before they have sex. Most women have always wanted good sex with one beloved man rather than a large number of partners, and many men are also getting tired of "recreational" sex. Men crave love and affection as much as women do, although some might find it a little more difficult to admit this out loud.

Sexually exclusive relationships and earlier marriages are on the rise, and I think many women will welcome this.

Some women are not ready for or do not want to make a lifetime commitment to one man. Yet some people are taking the position that you can no longer safely have a sexual relationship outside of a monogamous long-term relationship or marriage.

That is not true. You do not have to forgo sex for reasons of safety. You can remain sexually active if you choose to, and you can do this safely if you are willing to make some concessions to your health and your future.

But in order to eliminate the risk of AIDS without giving up romance, you have to be armed with scientifically accurate information about AIDS and how it is transmitted through sex.

3

AIDS: The Disease

AIDS is a viral infection that attacks the body's immune system and cripples the afflicted individual's ability to fight off certain illnesses and cancers, so that eventually he or she dies. You might have seen the virus referred to as HTLV-III or HTLV-III/LAV, and now it is called HIV, which stands for "human immunodeficiency virus," its newest and probably permanent scientific name.*

To avoid confusion, I have referred to the germ either as the "AIDS virus" or as HIV.

The AIDS virus is a slow retrovirus which may lie "dormant," which means quietly "sleeping," in your body for a long time.† Sometimes the AIDS virus begins to make a

---

* HTLV-III are the initials for Human T Lymphotropic Virus Type III, which is what American discoverers called the AIDS virus. The French, who found it at the same time, named it LAV or Lymphadenopathy Associated Virus. HIV is the new official scientific name for the AIDS virus which you will see more and more.

† Scientific References, Group V: AIDS Disease.

person ill within as short a time as six months after he has been infected, and at other times it may not become active for years or perhaps forever. AIDS is a new disease which scientists have studied only for six years. Therefore no one knows yet *how long* the AIDS virus can remain inactive, or "latent," * without causing any signs or symptoms of illness. We know for certain that the AIDS virus can lie dormant for at least seven years before actively attacking the victim. Although the natural history of AIDS is as yet unknown, we do know that each year more asymptomatic carriers become ill. Therefore infectious disease experts believe that the latency, or inactive, period might actually turn out to be much longer in some people, and it could be ten or more years before the infected person comes down with AIDS or with AIDS-related disease. Because the disease is so "slow" and so new, we still don't know, and we can't possibly know for another fifty years or more (i.e., for a full life span) whether all people who are infected will eventually die of AIDS, but the chances are that some are resistant or may even have a natural immunity.

As far as we know today, a person who becomes infected is infectious to others through blood, sex, and pregnancy and remains so, presumably for the rest of his or her life, but there may be long periods in the beginning stages of the disease where there are absolutely no external signs or symptoms of illness.

Between the moment of infection and the first appearance of AIDS symptoms the infected person is known as a *"healthy" carrier.*

The term "healthy" can be misleading, and it is extremely important for you to realize that men and women who are "healthy" carriers of the AIDS virus actually have an HIV infection and can infect their sexual partners.

* *Latent* is a medical term that means that a disease process is quiet but may break out at any time to make you ill, somewhat like an IOU note that can be collected whenever the person wants his money. *Dormant* and *inactive* mean the same thing.

Sex, blood, and pregnancy are the main pathways by which the AIDS virus is passed from person to person, but it has also been transmitted through breast milk and through organ transplants from infected donors. A few people have also become infected by being splashed by contaminated blood or other body fluids of AIDS patients and carriers.

This will make sense to you if you understand that the virus infects a certain kind of white blood cell called a T4-helper lymphocyte,* and also other kinds of white blood cells. Certain of these cells have the ability to move in and out of any of the moist organs of the human body. They easily pass in and out of blood vessels, and they can also move through the walls of organs such as the stomach, the lungs, and the heart.

These mobile virus-laden white blood cells are therefore present in the fluids and secretions and body tissues of infected persons, "healthy" carriers as well as those who are actually ill with AIDS or with AIDS-related diseases.†

But happily, while the virus-laden cells seem to "float" through any moist substance, *unbroken skin* of the dry kind acts as a barrier. Since the AIDS virus needs moisture to survive, it probably just dies on dry skin without doing any harm, unless it can find a nice wet entrance point into your body. It is not known exactly how long the AIDS virus can stay alive on a dry surface. Some studies suggest that the survival time could be as long as forty-eight hours.‡

---

* The T4 lymphocyte is also called a "helper" lymphocyte, in contrast to the T8 lymphocyte which is a "suppressor" lymphocyte. The most mobile of the white blood cells infected by this germ are *macrophages* and *monocytes*, but the lymphocytes also can pass in and out of blood vessels to get to the site of an infection when they are needed.

† Acquired Human Immunodeficiency Infection is a slowly progressing disease and before the illness becomes severe enough to be called AIDS the patient usually has numerous nonfatal symptoms. This stage of the disease used to be called ARC or AIDS-Related Complex. Now some doctors are referring to these complaints simply as the earlier stages of HIV infection.

‡ Although HIV can survive for forty-eight hours or even more in the laboratory, infectious disease specialists believe that in real life this is not the way the virus is transmitted from person to person. For all practical purposes, if you are going

Since so far not a single infection has been documented in household members who share bathroom facilities or who use the same telephone, dishes, and towels with AIDS carriers and AIDS patients, it is therefore the current consensus of scientific opinion that it is *perfectly safe to have close social, work, school, and family contact* with "healthy" carriers of the AIDS virus and with patients with AIDS and persons with AIDS-related conditions. However there are some disturbing recent reports that some family members who cared for sick AIDS patients were exposed to their infected secretions and became infected, so we have not heard the last word on this matter.

You will understand what I have to say about safe sex later on if you keep in mind that the AIDS virus on a dry surface is like a fish out of water and soon dies. And, although it is incredibly hardy and resistant to the body's own defenses and to medicines when it is inside the body, once it is outside the virus is very fragile and defenseless and can easily be killed by scrubbing with soap and water and by mild disinfectants like rubbing alcohol.

Therefore according to all the scientific evidence we have so far, all "dry" sexual practices are safe with anyone, but "wet sex," by which I mean erotic activities that involve the mingling of your body fluids with your partner's, or his infected body fluids coming into contact with the moist skin (or *mucous membranes*) that cover your genitals, is known to be extremely dangerous with carriers of the AIDS virus.*

This same thing is true about all sexually transmitted diseases (STDs). You will not catch syphilis or herpes by having dinner and going dancing with a syphilitic man or with a man who has an open herpes sore on his penis. Only by going to bed with him or by receiving a blood transfusion from him will you risk contracting the disease.

---

* *AIDS: Facts and Issues.* Victor Gong, M.D., and Norman Rudnick, editors, Rutgers Press, 1985.

---

to get AIDS, the chances are at least 97 percent that it will be from having sex with an infected partner or through infected blood.

THE LONG LATENCY PERIOD IS DANGEROUS

The AIDS virus belongs to a unique family of viruses called retroviruses. When these viruses infect one of the host's cells, they don't just sit there quietly like some other germs do. They actually take over control of the cell's metabolic machinery and exploit it to reproduce themselves.* One of the most dangerous features of retroviruses for human beings is that they can "sleep" quietly in the cells they have invaded for years and years and cause no visible problem. Then at some point, they become activated and make you ill. With the AIDS virus this can be six months to perhaps as much as a decade or more later.

You may be familiar with the herpes virus,† which also has a long period of latency, although it is a different kind of sexually transmitted virus. Over 90 percent of the citizens of this country are infected with lip herpes‡ from childhood on. This bug lies quietly dormant for years at a time, hiding out within some nerve cells that are connected to your lips without doing anything much, and by all appearances there is nothing wrong with you. Then when you get too much sun or you are under stress, or for no apparent reason at all, the herpes I virus becomes active and you break out with a nasty blister on your lip. It takes

* Retroviruses are equipped with an enzyme called reverse transcriptase, which gives them the ability to make a "genetic copy" of themselves which can survive in the host cell nucleus. Eventually this copy can "force" the infected host cell, for example a T4 lymphocyte, to reproduce more AIDS viruses until the lymphocyte finally dies. Then each AIDS virus emerges and takes over a new lymphocyte and repeats the cycle.

† The herpes virus that causes sores on the lips is classified as herpes simplex virus type I, which is closely related to herpes simplex virus II, or herpes genitalis, which has gotten very bad press because it causes genital herpes.

‡ Herpes simplex virus lies dormant in a special part of the *trigeminal nerve*, which supplies the face with sensation. When it is activated, new herpes virus is synthesized in the nerve cells and travels along the nerve fiber where it connects to the lip cells. There it reproduces further and develops a fever blister.

your immune system about ten days to put herpes back in its place and somewhat less if you are treated with drugs like *Acylovir*.* But the herpes virus doesn't die, it just re-treats into the trigeminal nerve cell or, in the case of herpes II, into special nerve cells that connect to your genitals, until your defenses are down again and then it zaps you once more.

Another unfortunate difference between herpes and AIDS is that you do not usually get herpes from a man if you kiss him unless he has an open blister on his lip and you don't get genital herpes if you have sex with him unless his infection is in the active phase. But if he is infected with HIV, even if he is not ill and is in the "healthy" carrier or dormant stage, you can definitely become infected from having sex with him even though he has no open sores or any other physical symptoms, since his secretions are swarming with AIDS-infected cells and free AIDS virus.

Most carriers are young, appear perfectly healthy, and are sexually active and fertile, just like herpes carriers. The only way you or a doctor can possibly tell if a man is a carrier is by knowing if he has been exposed to the AIDS virus and by the results of the AIDS antibody tests.

This is why the AIDS test is so crucial for your protection. AIDS testing, if properly used, can virtually eliminate the risks of your becoming infected with AIDS. But our educational programs have been abysmal and in many communities there is no access to affordable and anonymous AIDS testing, even for those who want to find out if they are infected.

EXPOSURE AND INFECTION

When I was testifying before a Congressional Committee on AIDS in April 1987, I was asked to comment on Mayor Koch's† objection to testing: "Why take the test if you al-

* *Acylovir* is probably the most effective anti-herpes drug available to date.
† Mr. Koch, the Mayor of New York City, is a strong antitest advocate.

ready know you've been exposed?" by which he seemed to be implying that exposure and infection are identical.

I explained that many people think that *exposure* to AIDS and *infection* with AIDS are the same thing.

But this is *wrong!* Do not be misled!

The difference between *exposure* to and *infection* with the AIDS virus is just like the difference between exposure to and infection with any other infectious disease, for example German measles. If one of your child's classmates comes down with German measles, your child has been *exposed* to the German measles virus (rubella), because the infected child has breathed virus-laden droplets into the commonly shared air of the classroom. Some of the children who have been exposed to German measles by inhaling the contaminated air will become infected, but others will not. Some infected children actually become ill, others become "asymptomatic" carriers. So you wait for the *incubation period* to pass. In the meantime although your child is not ill, he may be a highly contagious German measles carrier. You should not let him near your pregnant friends, who might give birth to a malformed baby if they are not immune and if they become infected. If he gets symptoms of German measles, a rash, swollen glands, and a fever, you put him to bed and make him as comfortable as you can, while the disease takes its course.

If he does not become ill in three weeks, you sigh with relief that *exposure* has not resulted in a rubella infection, and he can go near pregnant women again.

After a person is infected with German measles, he or she does not become a lifelong measles carrier. In fact, one acquires a long period of immunity against German measles, which is a good thing for girls because they don't have to worry about their baby when they get pregnant later. Unfortunately, once you are infected with the HIV virus not only do you become an AIDS carrier for life, but it is not known if anyone develops effective immunity. One thing is very fortunate, however. AIDS is not an airborne disease like flu or measles, spread by virus contained in little droplets of moisture exhaled with each breath by the infected person, and it is not nearly as contagious as chicken pox. The AIDS virus is transmitted from person to person primarily by blood, sex, and pregnancy from persons infected with AIDS and these are the only exposures you must avoid, literally, "like the plague."

Similarly, exposure to AIDS and infection with the AIDS virus are quite different. In fact, if you know that you have not been exposed it makes absolutely no sense for you to take the test. Testing is only for people who suspect they may have been exposed to enable them to determine if their exposure has resulted in infection.

You have *not* been exposed if you used a public telephone that has been used by an AIDS carrier, or if an infected person swam in your pool.*

But you could very well have been exposed to AIDS if you have had sex with a high-risk male or with a known AIDS carrier or an AIDS patient. If you have shared a hypodermic needle while using drugs, you most probably have been *exposed* to the AIDS virus and you should definitely have yourself tested to see if you've actually been *infected*.

If you have had sexual intercourse with a promiscuous man, especially if he is from a high-risk area or if he likes to have sex with high-risk women such as prostitutes, or if you have had sexual encounters with strangers in the past ten years, you cannot tell if you have been exposed but the chances that you were *infected* are still extremely small. But you might want to be tested just to find out if you have been infected just to be sure you are not going to give AIDS to your next lover.

If you received a blood transfusion between 1976 and 1984, or if you have had artificial insemination from a stranger donor during those years, the chances that you have been exposed are also extremely remote, but why not get tested and be certain?

* Chlorine kills the AIDS virus.

If you have been in a monogamous relationship or even if you have had sex with one or more "safe" or "ultrasafe" men (see Chapter 4), there is really not much reason for you to worry about exposure or to take the test. And although the risk of infection of drug-free American heterosexual males has doubled each year since 1976, in the country as a whole it's still only one in thirty thousand or less in 1987.* So you can see that even if you went to bed with a stranger last weekend, the chances are very small. *But please don't do it again.*

If you are obsessing about having caught AIDS from a sexual encounter with a handsome stranger on your vacation eight years ago you might just be feeling a little guilty —but by all means take the test. You will most probably find out that you are perfectly healthy. It is easy and inexpensive and if you can take the test at an alternative testing site which gives it anonymously, no one need ever know. (Testing will be explained in Chapter 4.) This is hardly necessary for medical reasons but it's good for your peace of mind.

The basic strategy for protecting yourself from AIDS is simple—*eliminate the risks of becoming infected by avoiding exposure.* If you cannot, or if you choose for any reason to expose yourself, then do the best you can to *reduce the risks of infection.*

THE SIGNS AND SYMPTOMS OF AIDS

Many people worry about being infected if they have swollen glands or fever or if they get any blemishes on their skin because one reads all kinds of things about the symptoms of AIDS. It is entirely unnecessary for you to torture yourself with worry because if you have any suspicious signs or symptoms that are due to aids, you will also have *antibodies*

* Scientific References, Group I: The Epidemiology of AIDS.

for AIDS in your blood, which will show up on the AIDS
test. Just get tested and find out.

It is difficult to understand the disease because patients
with AIDS suffer from innumerable symptoms and signs
and medical problems and succumb to a great variety of
different illnesses. This will make sense to you only if you
understand some basic scientific facts about the body's immune system.

Although we are not aware of this, we are constantly
being attacked by an invisible swarm of germs — viruses,
bacteria, protozoa, and microscopic fungi from the outside
— which would make us ill if our defenses didn't protect
us. We are also continually under the threat of being de-
stroyed by some of our own body cells, which can become
cancerous if they are not carefully monitored by the internal security forces of our bodies. Human beings survive
these internal and external enemies because we have
evolved an incredibly complex and highly effective defense
system. Under normal circumstances, we live in perfect
balance with our would-be attackers.

Our immune system is organized like the U.S. Department of Defense in that it is similarly made up of several
branches of specialized forces. Your armed forces include
(a) the *mechanical* barriers against bacterial invasion provided by the skin and the mucous membranes that line the
openings to your body, (b) a *chemical* warfare department
that produces special substances like interferon and other
agents in your tears, your saliva, and like the acid in your
stomach, which attack any germs that try to gain entrance
into your body through these routes, and (c) the most
sophisticated and important branch of all — the *immune
system.*

The immune system protects you when a germ or other
foreign invader gets past the outer mechanical and chemical defenses and actually invades your body. The immune
system also monitors your own cells so they don't get out
of hand and become malignant and destroy you.

We are born with certain inherited immune defenses,

but our survival depends most of all on our ability to *acquire* immunity to each of the hundreds of new viruses, bacteria, fungi, and protozoa which attack us.

The cornerstone of the body's ability to acquire immunity to new germs are certain white blood cells — macrophages, monocytes, and most important, various kinds of *lymphocytes.* Some of these cells, especially the macrophages, are extremely mobile and constantly circulate around the body, patrolling for foreign invaders. If they find one, they capture it and communicate with the appropriate B lymphocytes to generate specific immune defenses.

There are many different kinds of lymphocytes, each of which has a different and important function. The T-helper lymphocytes are crucial to the proper functioning of the immune system. Working as a team with the macrophages, they have the ability to "read" the structure of each of the thousands of microorganisms that try to invade us and of each unwelcomed foreign substance that is introduced to our bodies.

T-helper lymphocytes * recognize each new invader and become *programmed on the first encounter to recognize it forever after.* After the system has once been sensitized to a particular germ, the T4 lymphocyte will see to it that another kind of lymphocyte, the B *lymphocyte,* makes a specific antibody, which is a kind of poison designed to kill just that particular germ anytime it tries to invade you again. To do this lymphocytes are equipped with superb intelligence and memory functions. In general, any infectious microbe that you have ever encountered since you were six months old will be greeted by the immune system's specific antibody that will destroy it if it ever tries to get you again. Thus if you've had German measles, chicken pox, or mumps as a child and your immune system is working

---

* T-helper lymphocytes are the same as T4-lymphocytes, and regulate the entire immune system. T8-lymphocytes are *suppressor* cells, which make sure that the B-lymphocytes, which make antibodies, don't overdo it.

normally, you will never again become ill with these diseases. Every time you are exposed to measles or chicken pox or mumps virus, and the chances are good that you will be, the macrophage–T-helper lymphocyte team "remembers." Instantly these cells help the B-lymphocytes to make great quantities of specific mumps or German measles or chicken pox antibodies, which zap the virus before it can get a foothold in your body and make you (or your infant when you are pregnant) ill.

Each different virus "likes" certain kinds of cells and is not interested in others. For example the polio virus only infects certain motor nerve cells, while the cells that line your nose and throat specifically attract the virus that gives you the common cold.

HIV attaches itself to and invades any cell that has a T4 receptor on its surface.* These are found on T4-helper lymphocytes, and also on certain nerve cells, macrophages, monocytes, and on some other cells as well. Unfortunately the AIDS virus has a special affinity for and a tendency to invade and damage *T4-helper lymphocytes*, which play *a key role in regulating and controlling the entire acquired immune system.*

Just think how devilish the AIDS virus is. Some of the white blood cells it invades are extremely mobile because they are supposed to wander all over your body and into all your secretions to look for and capture invaders, and to get to injured places of the body. But once you are infected it is this very mobility that enables the AIDS virus to find new hosts, and AIDS is often transmitted from one person to another by "hitching a ride" on those busy little wandering cells that contain viral "time bombs."

AIDS patients become ill from and then die of numerous unusual infections and odd cancers that usually don't hurt people because a normal immune system has no trouble defending against them. But certain infections take advan-

* *Receptor sites* are special "doors" on the cell's surface to which certain substances that are needed by that cell have the "key." Each kind of cell has a different cluster of receptor sites.

tage of the opportunity provided by the sabotaging of the victim's immune system, and for this reason they are called opportunistic infections.

The human body does not give up easily and it tries desperately albeit vainly to defend itself against the AIDS virus. When the AIDS virus invades the victim's body, the immune system responds in its usual way by making large quantities of AIDS antibodies against the AIDS virus. Even though this is unfortunately ineffective against the germ, the production of AIDS antibodies usually continues until the patient is exhausted and near the end of his or her life. The only good thing about the AIDS antibody is that it leaves a trail that can be detected by the antibody tests and this is what enables us to find out if a person is a carrier long before there are any laboratory or clinical findings of the illness.

The AIDS antibody is not only ineffective against the HIV virus, but something even worse happens. HIV knocks out the crucial T4 lymphocytes, and thereby damages the patient's immune system so badly that it loses its ability to make any antibodies against certain dangerous *new* invaders. This leaves AIDS patients without any *cellular defenses*, and they are sitting ducks for opportunistic infections and cancers, to which they eventually succumb.

The first or early signs of AIDS — weight loss, fatigue, low-grade fever, and swollen lymph nodes — are not specific for AIDS. They are also seen in many other diseases as well, such as mononucleosis, and other Barr-Epstein virus infections, or for that matter, any low-grade infection. But with patients who have AIDS, the symptoms don't go away or they constantly recur, so that the patient never feels perfectly well again. The pattern of the disease varies widely. In many cases the disease progresses slowly over the years but in some cases it develops quickly. Scientists do not yet understand why this is so.

Not every patient who goes on to develop AIDS experiences the early symptoms that were described above. Some gradually become sicker and sicker, but others come down with an opportunistic infection before having experienced any sort of medical problem, and it is not unusual for a patient who appears perfectly healthy to suddenly become desperately ill and die.

The earliest sign of HIV infection is a self-limiting* mononucleosislike illness called *acute HIV* infection which some patients experience two weeks to six months after exposure. The symptoms include fever, sweating, swollen glands, stiff neck, and sometimes a scattered red rash. This shows that the body is trying to fight off the virus with fever, by "fixating" it in the skin and, most important, by making AIDS antibodies. Some persons seroconvert silently, so that there are often no physical signs of acute AIDS infection at all, and the only evidence that the person has HIV infection is that he or she starts to make AIDS antibodies which can be detected by the AIDS tests. After seroconversion nothing else happens for six months or seven years or forever. This is the "healthy" carrier or latency stage of the disease.

Sometimes, later, while the patient is still to all outward appearances "healthy," the AIDS virus begins to deplete and destroy the T4 helper lymphocytes. At this stage the patient's blood shows a drop in the T4 lymphocytes relative to the other kinds of lymphocytes.

As the disease slowly progresses, the patient may develop swollen glands in the neck, groin, or armpits, and blood tests now will show that the immune system is getting much worse. Not only are his T4 lymphocytes becoming fewer in number, but those that remain are now also damaged. This phase of the disease had been called ARC, which stands for AIDS-Related Complex, but as doctors began to understand the progression of the disease better, they began to refer to various stages and forms of HIV infection. When early physical signs begin to appear — persistent fever and night sweats, swollen lymph glands,

---

* The common cold is a self-limiting illness which runs its course and then clears up without doing much damage.

fatigue, depression, irritability, headaches, and unexplained weight loss — the syndrome is now classified as AIDS-related constitutional disease.

The patient is now gradually losing the ability to defend himself against opportunistic infections, and previously healthy individuals are now likely to have long, lingering colds; thrush (a yeast infection that causes white creamy patches to form on the tongue, mouth, throat, and anorectal area); persistent or recurrent diarrhea; coughing due to a rare kind of pneumonia (Pneumonia carinii); easy bruising of the skin; and strange-looking rashes and bumps on the skin that can appear on any part of the body.

The skin problems are often the manifestations of Kaposi's sarcoma,* and have so far mostly been observed in homosexual males with AIDS. The appearance of these dreaded painless red or purple spots and bumps heralds the presence of this rapidly progressive and fatal cancer.

The AIDS virus also attacks the brain, and in later stages AIDS patients may suffer from *AIDS dementia*, which is characterized by confusion, depression, irrational behavior, and signs of spinal cord and nerve damage such as double vision, stumbling, weakness, and numbness. Unless the doctor knows about AIDS, these neurological symptoms can be misdiagnosed as a psychological problem.

Uncontrollable herpes sores which erupt all over the patient's body; Pneumocystis carinii pneumonitis, which causes a chronic dry hacking cough and shortness of breath; other infections which cause debilitating diarrhea and respiratory problems that we don't see in well-nourished people with normal immune systems; and a group of unusual cancers and blood diseases often occur in the later stages of AIDS. These are called opportunistic diseases, and the patient usually dies of one of these.

---

* Kaposi's sarcoma is a rare form of cancer only seen in persons with defective immune systems, including extremely old patients whose immune system has deteriorated, patients who have had radiation for cancer; and organ recipients who receive drugs to suppress their immune response so that their bodies do not reject their newly transplanted kidney or heart.

Table 4   *The Stages and Symptoms of AIDS, or HIV, Infection*

STAGE I — ACUTE AIDS, OR HIV, INFECTION

A. **Blood Studies:** Antibodies to HIV virus present in patient's blood, presumably for life.

B. **Clinical Features:** Some persons infected with HIV have a transient mononucleosis-like *illness* one week to several months after they were infected. This consists of fever, fatigue, swollen glands, and in some patients a rash. A few develop aseptic meningitis, with stiff neck, vomiting, and headache. These symptoms disappear in a few days or weeks and indicate that seroconversion is taking place.

STAGE II — ASYMPTOMATIC AIDS, OR HIV, INFECTION

A. **Blood Studies:** Reveal progressive depletion of T4-helper lymphocytes as compared with the T8-suppressor lymphocytes.

B. **Clinical Features:** The "healthy" carrier stage of AIDS. The patient has no visible signs of illness.

STAGE III — PROGRESSIVE GENERALIZED LYMPHADENOPATHY (FORMERLY CALLED AIDS-RELATED COMPLEX, OR ARC)

A. **Blood Studies:** Reveal further destruction of T4-helper lymphocytes.

B. **Clinical Features:** Swollen lymph glands on neck or groin or armpits, etc. Otherwise the patient feels fine.

STAGE IV — AIDS OR OTHER HIV DISEASES

A. **Blood Studies:** Now reveal severe destruction and depletion of lymphocytes.

B. **Clinical Features:** Four stage IV or AIDS syndromes have been recognized.

1. *Constitutional Disease.* The patient feels depressed and fatigued, and has persistent or recurrent fever, night sweats, weight loss, swollen glands, diarrhea, and "wasting."

2. *Neurological Disease.* AIDS *dementia,* which consists of irrational behavior and loss of judgment; various neurological problems such as loss of balance and double vision, and numbness and/or weakness of the arms and/or legs.

3. *Opportunistic Infections and Cancers.* The patient develops one or more infections with certain viruses, bacteria, fungi, or protozoa to which persons with a normal immune system are resistant, and/or some invasive cancers which are either very mild or do not occur in persons with adequate cell-mediated immunity.

   These diseases produce a variety of chronic or recurring medical *signs and symptoms,* including: fever, respiratory difficulties, meningitis, persistent diarrhea, skin bumps and rashes, fatigue, depression, bizarre behavior, and general wasting.

The Most Common Opportunistic Diseases Seen in the United States Are:

- *Pneumocystis carinii pneumonia (PCP):* Persistent dry, hacking cough and progressive shortness of breath.

- *Severe candida (also called thrush, or yeast infection):* Creamy white patches in the mouth; the tongue; other parts of the gut, including the ano-rectal area; and the airways. (Vaginal thrush by itself is *not* a sign of AIDS.)

- *Disseminated herpes simplex:* Large patches of herpes sores erupt on all parts of the body, including the ano-rectal area. (A fever blister is *not* a sign of AIDS.)

- *Kaposi's sarcoma:* Mostly seen in homosexual men, a cancer of the blood vessels that causes the patient to break out in *red to purple* blotches and/or bumps on all parts of the body and also on various internal organs.)

- *Non-Hodgkins lymphomas:* Primary lymphoma of the brain — headache, neurological symptoms. Other lymphomas: tumors on various internal organs, fever, swollen glands.

Rarer Opportunistic Infections. The prevalence of these differs in different areas of the country:

- *Progressive multifocal leukoencephalopathy* — neurologic symtpoms.

- *Chronic cryptosporidiosis* — meningitis, general illness.

- *Toxoplasmosis* — headache, confusion, vomiting.

- *Strongyloidosis* (extraintestinal) — general illness.

- *Iosporiasis* — chronic diarrhea.

- *Cryptococciosis* — diarrhea.

- *Histoplasmosis* — pneumonia, general illness.

- *Mycobacterial infections with M. Avium Intracellulare or M. Kansaii* — pneumonia, general illness.

4. *Other Medical Problems Seen in Patients with AIDS.* The CDC also list the following infections and cancers as being unusually common and/or virulent in patients with AIDS-related defects in cellular immunity: oral hairy leukoplakia, Barr-Epstein virus, tuberculosis, multidermatosal herpes zoster (severe shingles), hepatitis B, salmonella acteremia, and certain solid cancers of the tongue and ano-rectal areas.

This table is based on the current official classification system which was first proposed by the CDC in 1986, and on the forthcoming revision. The term "AIDS" had been used only for patients who have the opportunistic diseases specified for Stage IV, subgroup 3. However, the CDC has now determined that patients who have severe wasting (1), or neurological disease (2) also have AIDS.

CHILDREN AND AIDS

The first baby infected with AIDS while in the uterus of its infected mother was reported in 1983, although cases have since been traced back as early as 1979. In recent years AIDS in children has been increasing steadily so that by 1987 over 500 cases have been reported to the CDC (United States Centers for Disease Control), and of these 322 have died. But there are probably many more that have never been reported. Although children with AIDS currently constitute only around 1 percent of the total AIDS cases in the United States, experts are predicting that the number of children born with AIDS will now increase sharply as the disease *spreads among women of child-bearing age*. The CDC estimates that unless the spread to women is halted, 4000 children will die in the next five years.*

According to one excellent study done by Drs. Rubinstein and Bernstein at the Albert Einstein Medical College in a poor section of New York City, "the reasons that a child under twelve years of age will get AIDS are, in the order of frequency: 1. the mother is infected with AIDS; 2. the father is infected with AIDS; 3. the child received infected blood; 4. the child was sexually abused by an infected man; 5. the child was exposed to contaminated needles at home."

The doctors who reported this study found that "children of I.V. drug abusing mothers and/or fathers and children of bisexual fathers comprised a majority of all patients. All the mothers who were married to high-risk men were positive for HTLV-III antibodies. In 70 percent of all cases the mothers acquired the disease through intravenous drug abuse; in 23 percent of the cases the disease was contracted by the mother through sexual contact with a bisexual or through promiscuity." The mothers then gave the disease to their children.

---

* Scientific References, Group II: AIDS in Children.

One case which particularly troubled me, because it might have been prevented if only the blood banks had excluded male homosexual donors before the AIDS test became available, was that of a woman who became infected with the AIDS virus when she received a transfusion of contaminated blood after the delivery. She subsequently breast-fed her baby for six weeks and the baby became infected.*

Another case which is horrifying in its brutality was that of a five-year-old boy who became ill with AIDS. The doctors reported that they "felt that the child had not contracted the disease through intrauterine transmission." Intensive investigation finally revealed that this boy was sexually abused by his AIDS stricken bisexual father. Another equally shocking case described by the same investigators was "a seven-year-old girl whose AIDS infection was caused by the use of contaminated drug needles by family members on the child."

SIGNS AND SYMPTOMS OF AIDS IN BABIES AND CHILDREN

Some babies who are infected before they are born have a peculiar type of facial appearance† which indicates that they were infected during the first three months of their development. Many are born a little underweight and some have swollen glands and other early symptoms of HIV infection. But most infected infants look perfectly healthy and the doctor can only tell for sure that the baby is infected by performing the AIDS test, after six months, and again one year later, after *his infected mother's* AIDS antibodies have disappeared from his bloodstream.

* Newborn infants, especially premature ones, are especially vulnerable to infection and any blood transfusions should be very carefully screened for AIDS.
† Some investigators reported at the Third International Conference on AIDS, which was held in Washington, D.C., in June 1987, that they observed abnormally formed or "dysmorphic" facial structures in a small number of babies born with HIV infection.

The blood and the immune system of babies that are born with AIDS shows similar abnormalities to those described for adults, and the average age when the baby begins to show signs of illness is around six months. The earliest onset of symptoms of AIDS in one study was observed in a six-week-old patient, while the longest disease-free period was around two years. Experts in this area feel that any child who develops symptoms of AIDS after he or she has reached the age of two should be investigated carefully to make sure that the infection is not due to sexual abuse, contaminated blood needles, or infected blood products.

The most common health problems of children with AIDS or pre-AIDS are recurrent infections, and infections that seem to last much longer than they do in other children. AIDS kids also tend to get much sicker with every infection. Persistent and recurrent mouth lesions (thrush) and the failure to thrive are also very common, as are swollen lymph glands, persistent or recurrent diarrhea, and enlargement of the salivary glands. A unique and common finding in children with AIDS is chronic lymphoid pneumonitis. This is a chronic chest problem, not quite as bad as pneumonia, which is caused by Pneumocystis carinii. The children cough and have difficulty breathing and have fevers, and nothing seems to cure them.

Toward the final stages of the illness, children infected by the AIDS virus develop the same sort of unusual infections that adults do. When these infections occur in the first year of life the child seldom survives beyond the second year, even though he or she may be actively treated. Some children who are born infected do not develop the late stages of AIDS and the opportunistic infections until the age of seven.

4

Prevention: Condoms Are Not Safe Enough

You are being bombarded by conflicting, contradictory, and confusing statements issued by physicians, public health experts, sex educators, politicians, religious leaders, do-gooders, and do-badders about "safe sex," "unsafe sexual practices," "protected sex." You have heard: "Healthcare workers are safe with AIDS patients," and "The blood supply is safe."

Please don't believe it just because you read it in the newspapers and don't believe everything you hear from your friends, your minister, your congressman, or even your doctor. Especially don't apply everything you hear about "safe sex" to yourself because most of the educational programs are mainly for the benefit of the high-risk homosexual community. Women's health has *not* had a high priority in AIDS educational campaigns so far. So use your own head and judge everything you hear for yourself. Remember that relying on inaccurate or incomplete information and/or bad advice could be dangerous to your health!

I would like to see T.V. spots that say: "Women, the men you are dating are not likely to be infected unless they shoot drugs or are bisexual. Do not have sex with such a high-risk man. If you are not sure, *hold out* until he is tested and cleared!" It is maddening that this obvious point is not being made in the public educational campaigns.

Please keep that message in mind when you see those male-oriented "wear your rubbers" ads. Not so long ago we were seeing "public service" spots on T.V.* that showed a beautiful woman with a condom in her hand saying with a sweet smile, "I'd rather be safe than dead." If she relies on a condom instead of the test, she could die if some infected fluid from his moist pubic hair touches her genitalia.

Think about that when you read some of the books that they are giving to the adolescents, some of which give young people dangerous advice: "A condom is the best known prevention against AIDS." † The books and most of the sex education courses that I have checked out fail to mention that *avoidance of exposure* is a preferable strategy for this age group. You may read in "female"-oriented books, "Assert yourself, ask him to use a condom." *Nonsense! He* wants intercourse so badly that he might be willing to use a condom. *You* should *really* assert yourself by making *him* take the responsibility for finding out his AIDS status. Say *No* to him until he is tested and cleared. (But then volunteer to go with him and have yourself tested too.)

You are not likely to get AIDS from a toilet seat or from eating in a restaurant where the cook is gay. That is like worrying that you will be killed by a brick falling off a building. You should worry about *real* dangers. Virtually the *only* way those of you who will die of AIDS will catch it is by having sex with an infected man. Therefore, reducing the risks of exposure is not good enough for you or your daughter. The story is different when you are in a relation-

---

* Advertisements (sponsored by the New York Health Department) implying that sex with condoms is safe, were appearing in New York City on public television up to June 1987.

† *Sex, Drugs, and AIDS*, by Oralee Wachter, Bantam Books, 1987.

ship with a man who has AIDS or is a carrier. In that case, of course, you should try to reduce the risks. But otherwise *eliminating* the risks of sexual transmission of AIDS should clearly be the first-line strategy for women.

I cannot make the point strongly enough that at this time, women in this country by and large have not yet been exposed to the AIDS virus, and of those who have, only a very few have been infected. There is still time for the great majority of you to avoid getting AIDS.

I practice in New York City, which has the highest number of AIDS patients and the highest concentration of asymptomatic, or "silent,"* AIDS carriers in the world. A woman who has sex with a stranger in the New York metropolitan area is probably taking one hundred times the risk that her cousin from Wyoming is taking if she has sex with a local man.

Some of my women patients who have had casual sex were or could have been exposed to AIDS. I encourage everyone who has been exposed to be tested, and fortunately so far all my women patients have been negative. They have sighed with relief, thanked God that they have escaped—and determined that they would never again be so self-destructive as to risk their lives and their futures by allowing themselves to be exposed. The same goes for you. The chances that you have been exposed are still slim, and even if you have been exposed, there is every reason to believe that if you have yourself tested you too will find that you have escaped. *And it is vital that you keep it that way!*

DEGREES OF SEXUAL RISKS FOR AMERICAN WOMEN: 1987

You should be aware that there are three things that determine the degree of risk of contracting AIDS you are taking

---

* A person who is infected but has no visible symptoms of AIDS is called a "healthy" or "silent" or "asymptomatic" carrier of the HIV virus.

by going to bed with a particular man: (1) his AIDS *risk* status, (2) *where* he lives and makes love, and (3) *how* you make love together.

We have already discussed the most important item, whether or not he belongs to a high-risk group. You can only tell this from his sex and drug history. I would like to repeat that if he does not belong to a high-risk group, the chances that he is an AIDS carrier today are probably less than one in thirty thousand,* but if he is a male who belongs to one of the two high-risk groups, the possibility that he is infected is as high as up to seven out of ten (70 percent) in some places like New York, San Francisco, or Washington, D.C., which have the highest prevalence of AIDS in the country.

Men who are difficult to "read" because they are closed off and noncommunicative are now especially dangerous for women. If a man finds it hard to be open about sex, the AIDS test is the only safeguard for you. With this kind of man it is especially important that you volunteer to have yourself tested also.

LOCATION

Where he lives and where he makes love also make a difference in determining the chances that your new sexual partner is infected, although these are a lot less important than knowing if he belongs to a high- or low-risk group.

The AIDS virus is just beginning to leak out of the geographical high-risk centers and is much more heavily concentrated even in the heterosexual population in those areas. There is already a significant difference in the level of infection in various areas of the country. Communities where groups of homosexuals live attract bisexual men, many of whom are married and in "the closet," for homo-

---

* See Figure 4 which shows where there are many infected persons, and where the AIDS virus is still very rare.

Figure 4 LOCATION: Degrees of Risk

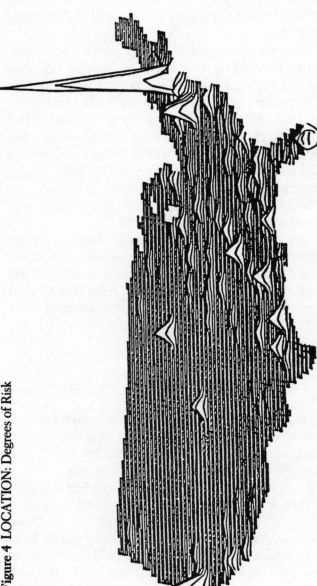

Three-dimensional representation of the county-specific prevalence of HIV infection in civilian applicants for military service from October 1985 to March 1986 (Walter Reed Institute of Research).

Source of the data: Robert R. Redfield, M.D., and Donald S. Burke, M.D., "Shadow on the Land: The Epidemiology of HIV Infection," *American Journal of Immunology*, 1987.

sexual interludes. The AIDS virus has become more prevalent in the surrounding heterosexual communities through "bridges" of women who have then had sex with these infected bisexual men.

The three-dimensional map indicates the prevalence of AIDS carriers in different regions of the country. The high risk areas are easy to pinpoint. If your man lives in or travels to San Francisco or New York and has sex there, he is five times more likely to be infected than if he stays put in Ohio or Montana or Wyoming.

Sailors who go on shore leave in Africa are dangerous. Men who visit prostitutes in high-risk cities (see Table 2 in Chapter 1) are also more likely to be carriers, but they are not as a group as highly infected as bisexuals and I.V. drug users.

Table 5 *MEN: Degrees of Risk*

HIGH-RISK MEN Do not have sex or have only safe "dry sex" with this man unless he has been tested and cleared and is in a monogamous relationship with you.

1. Bisexual and homosexual men—over 70% are infected in some areas.
2. I.V. drug users—up to 75% are infected in some areas.
3. Recipients of blood products:
   a. hemophiliacs—up to 80% of certain types of hemophiliacs have been infected in some locations. *
   b. men who have had transfusions between 1981 and 1984—now only one or two out of a million blood recipients are being infected. †
4. Promiscuous heterosexual men who have multiple sexual encounters with high-risk prostitutes or I.V. drug users, and/or with many women they do not know. Risk varies with location and with the number of exposures. Possibly between 0.1% and 0.5% have been infected.

MIDDLE-RISK MEN Better not to have sex with this man until he is tested; certainly wear condoms until you have been in a monogamous relationship with him for six months, or stick to safe dry sex.

1. A married man who has a pattern of monogamous relationships and who is currently not having sex with his wife.

---

* Scientific References, Group V: AIDS the Disease.
† Scientific References, Group VII: Transmission of AIDS by Infected Blood.

Table 5   *MEN: Degrees of Risk (cont.)*

2. Men who have had few sexual encounters (not with prostitutes). Risks not known, but probably less than 0.04%.

3. Men who live in or travel to high-risk areas (see Figure 4) are always more dangerous than those who do not live in or travel to high-risk areas.

LOW-RISK MEN   Sex with this man is probably safe, but until you are certain he is telling the truth and that he is not sleeping with anyone else, why not stick to safe dry sex or ask him to wear a condom and reduce the risk even further.

1. Men who have a pattern of long-lasting serial monogamous relationships.

2. Recently widowed men who had monogamous marriages and you are their first partner.

3. Someone you have known for a long time (perhaps you grew up with him) and are certain is not high risk.

4. Men who belong to reputable "AIDS free" clubs. ‡

SAFE MEN

1. A man who has been your steady, monogamous partner or husband for more than ten years.

2. A man who is your monogamous partner who has been tested and cleared.

‡ Because of the growing AIDS danger a number of privately funded and profit-making organizations have sprung up for single persons who are looking for safe relationships. These clubs require members to undergo repeated testing with screening tests. Usually these organizations are not interested in finding out whether you *have* AIDS, only whether you do *not* have AIDS. One such club pairs up people in three categories: (1) both are seronegative, (2) both are seropositive, (3) neither will take the test. You still can not have casual sex safely with a man who has an "AIDS-free" card, because he might have been exposed *after* he took his last test. You still have to get to know him and trust that he is decent and honest.

SAFE SEX TO SUICIDAL SEX

Abstaining from sex altogether is of course entirely safe. On the other hand, the highest-risk sexual practice, which I call "suicidal," is to have repeated unprotected sexual intercourse with an infected man or men.

But there are many degrees of risk between celibacy and suicidal sex which you should understand for your protection.

Using what we know about AIDS at this time, I prepared a list of sexual practices; it goes from sex that is *probably* safe to sex that carries the greatest risks, even with a partner whose AIDS status you do not know. The safety "ratings" used here are highly educated guesses, and are based on the facts as we know them today, but these estimates have not been confirmed, nor are they likely to be, because it is most difficult to sort out different sexual practices for scientific studies. So the advice given and the suggestions made must be read with the possibility of error in mind. However, I firmly believe that these suggestions and judgments are well founded in current scientific information, and taking into account the fact that one normally takes certain risks, when one travels, exercises, works, has children, etc., and the importance of love and sex in one's life, these assessments are reasonable and valid.

Table 6   *SEXUAL TRANSMISSION: Degrees of Risk*

1. *No Risks:* Celibacy, no sex at all. *100% safe.*

2. *Ultrasafe Sex:* No touching each other. *100% safe.* Talking sexy; sharing your sexual fantasies, sharing erotica; telephone sex.

3. *Safe Sex: Dry Sex: No exchanged body fluids. Probably 100% safe.* Caressing the dry parts of each other's bodies; masturbating in each other's presence but no physical contact.

4. *Low-Risk Sex: No mingling of infected body fluids. Probably not 100% safe but close.* Stimulation of each other's genitalia to orgasm without mingling of body fluids; vaginal, anal, or oral sex using a condom with a partner you have every reason to believe is not infected but whose AIDS status you are not certain of. (But watch out, these exciting experiences entail the danger of your being "swept away" by your passion into an unsafe sexual act.)

5. *High-Risk Sex: 10% to 30% possibility of infection if he is a carrier.* Vaginal or anal intercourse using condoms, with a high-risk male, or with a male who might have been exposed, or with a stranger whose exposure history you do not know. Oral sex with this kind of man could be just as risky.

6. *Suicidal Sex: 50% to 85% probability that you might become infected* with the AIDS virus if this is repeated, but you can catch AIDS on a *single exposure.* Unprotected vaginal, anal, or oral intercourse with a high-risk male or with a stranger, or with a known carrier.

HOW AIDS IS TRANSMITTED THROUGH SEX

Most sexual experiences involve some mingling of the partners' body fluids, as well as contact between the moist parts of their genitalia and body openings. The secretions and moist kind of skin of the person infected with the AIDS virus (including "healthy" HIV carriers as well as patients with AIDS and AIDS-related medical problems) contain the HIV virus and infected lymphocytes and macrophages that are loaded with the virus. AIDS virus and infected cells have been recovered from the blood, semen, vaginal secretions, saliva, tears, and breast milk of AIDS-infected persons. AIDS virus can be transmitted from person to person if the virus or some infected cells are able to enter the new victim's body.

The AIDS virus and AIDS-infected cells can enter your body only if they come in contact with your "wet" type of skin, or mucous membranes, which cover your mouth, nose, nipples, rectum, anus, and genital organs. These are the vulnerable entrance ports for the virus.

Probably *all* sexually transmitted diseases, including syphilis and genital herpes among others, not only AIDS, can enter your body only through moist places. The infected body fluids can also gain access directly into the next victim's blood stream through blood transfusions, or by way of an infected hypodermic needle, or perhaps even through little cuts or scrapes on the skin. But if you get some infected secretions, such as the seminal fluid of a man with AIDS on the unbroken dry kind of skin of your hand, there is "zero evidence" that the AIDS virus can gain entrance into your body or that you can become infected.

The female sexual organs are covered by moist, vulnerable mucous membranes that affords the virus an easy point of entrance into your body, should some infected lymphocytes or free virus particles land there.

The dry skin that covers the outside of your body is called "cornified" and is quite different from the moist mucous membrane that lines the openings to your body. Dry skin has a thin, tough, flexible layer of cornified material which protects the body from injury and dehydration. This dry kind of skin acts as a barrier to many germs, including HIV, and you won't get infected even if you get wet from walking in the rain or taking a shower with your lover. By contrast, the moist skin that lines your mouth, vagina, anus, and the opening of your nipples, where fluid loss is not a problem, does not have a protective cornified layer. But there are little pockets of lymphocytes which are supposed to guard the entrance parts of your body against invasion. The AIDS virus can gain entrance into your body through these moist mucous membranes to infect you. Scientists are not yet sure whether the virus and/or infected cells just pass through, or infect the host's lymphoid follicules, or get directly into the bloodstream through little nicks, or all of the above.

But remember, the AIDS virus can enter your body even if you do not have any skin injuries, right through your mucous membranes.*

Now let's look at how the AIDS virus can actually be transmitted in the course of various sexual activities.

During *vaginal intercourse* the man's infected preejaculatory secretions, the little drop of clear fluid that sometimes comes out of the tip of the man's penis when he is aroused but before he ejaculates, as well as his seminal fluid, are squirted into the woman's vulnerable wet vagina and can infect her. If the woman has the virus, her infected vaginal lubrications pour over the open moist entrance to the man's urethra (the small opening at the tip of the penis where the urine and semen emerge) and he can become infected through that route. Uncircumcised men might be more vulnerable than circumcised men because the glans (the scientific name for the head of the penis), which is covered by the foreskin when the penis is not erect, is

---

* AIDS: *Facts and Issues* by Victor Gong, M.D., and Norman Rudnick, editors, Rutgers Press, 1985.

covered with moist skin and this provides an additional passageway for the virus. The glans in circumcised males may become less penetrable to the AIDS virus and infected cells.

If the vaginal or penile skin has minute injuries or abrasions, which are very common, the likelihood of infection may be greatly increased because the infected fluids have direct access to the new host's bloodstream.

The same secretions are exchanged and the same moist membranes touch when a couple snuggles together after making love.

During *oral sex*, when a woman stimulates an infected man's penis orally (fellatio), the moist lining of the woman's mouth, her oral mucous membrane, is in contact with the wet infected opening of the man's urethra and also with his infected pre-ejaculatory fluids. If he ejaculates inside her mouth, she is also exposed to his semen, which has a high concentration of AIDS virus and infected cells.

The man is also at risk if he kisses, sucks, or licks an infected woman's genitalia (cunnilingus). His vulnerable wet mouth and tongue are exposed to her virus-laden genital secretions and the moist skin covering her vulva, which could be teeming with infected lymphocytes and/or free virus. The danger of transmission of the virus from fellatio and cunnilingus may be increased considerably if either have bleeding gums or little injuries in their mouths, which as you know are extremely common.

Anal intercourse is also dangerous, especially for the recipient. The anus was not designed for sexual purposes, and in contrast to the elastic, flexible, and lubricated vagina, it is tighter and harder to enter and more likely to be injured by penile penetration. The moist lining of the recipient's vulnerable anus and rectum is exposed to the same infected fluids as the vagina during vaginal intercourse, with the additional hazard that the anal skin and the thin, fragile mucous lining of the rectum is more likely to be traumatized or torn by hard penile thrusting.

The inserter is not without risk, because the vulnerable

moist parts of his penis make contact with the partner's anal lining and also with his or her feces, which may contain AIDS virus. But the danger apparently is less for him.

Kissing can theoretically transmit the AIDS virus and virus-laden lymphocytes from the infected partner's saliva to the healthy one's moist oral linings and directly into the bloodstream through any bleeding gums and mouth sores. But since lovers usually kiss during intercourse, who can tell if it's the kiss or the coitus which is transmitting the virus?

None of these sexual practices is safe with an infected person *with or without condoms* because his secretions and the moist parts of his body are loaded with living AIDS material, and these can get around and over a condom even if it does not break.

Scientists don't know why some people who have sex with seropositive partners become infected, while others, who engage in the same sexual practices, remain healthy.

It may be speculated that the *density* of the virus in the partner's body fluids is one factor. If your lover's semen contains a high concentration of AIDS virus particles and infected cells, you are probably more likely to become infected than if there are only a few.

Another element is that people vary in their susceptibility to the AIDS virus. Some people are just naturally more resistant to HIV than others. That is possibly why approximately 50 percent of babies of seropositive mothers become infected during pregnancy, and 50 percent don't.

You might hear that some sexual "perverted" practices such as homosexual sex, anal sex, or oral sex are "high risk" and *cause* AIDS. That is not true. As long as your partner is not a carrier of the AIDS virus his mucous membranes and his body fluids do not contain any harmful material and you cannot catch AIDS through any form of sexual activity with him.

Therefore it is nonsense to speak of "avoiding unsafe sexual practices." All sexual practices are safe with an uninfected man. *"Avoid infected partners!"* must be our slogan. No form of wet sex is free of risks with them and that is true with or without condoms.

I am not endorsing any of these practices. I have always maintained that one should never do anything sexually that does not feel good or right emotionally or physically. Your refusal should be based on moral or emotional or personal grounds, but you need not fear AIDS if your partner is not infected. (Safe sex and dangerous sex are described in Chapter 5.)

Finally, the risk of infection is directly related to the *number of partners* and the *number of sexual exposures* you have to infected men. In the case of AIDS, *less* is definitely better than more.

CONDOMS

Now I want to explain why I have been saying that condoms alone, especially when you do not know your partner, are not safe enough for women. This is most important for those of you who want to have children someday, and that certainly includes adolescents, who have their entire lives before them.

The simple truth is that while it is almost certain that condoms reduce the risks of infection, the level of protection that condoms confer when you have sex with an infected man is *not known*. We do know for certain, however, that it is by no means 100 percent!!! *

Many sexual health professionals like myself *wish* that condoms were the answer to the prevention of the heterosexual transmission of AIDS. That would really make things easy. If condoms were really safe, we would not need testing, with its complex legal and political problems. There would be no need to worry about civil rights infringements or health insurance problems of AIDS carriers, because we wouldn't need testing! We could return

* Scientific References, Group III: Condoms.

to the carefree days of riskless casual sex, except that we would use condoms. If condoms were really safe all we would need is an educational campaign urging people to use condoms whenever they have sex and free distribution of condoms to those who can not afford them.

But we can't allow ourselves to be misled by wishful thinking.

You may be hearing from pro-condom advocates that several scientific studies have definitely shown that under *laboratory conditions* the AIDS virus cannot pass through latex condoms. Test-tube studies have also shown that spermicides containing nonoxynol-9 inactivate the AIDS virus itself and the cells which carry the AIDS virus. All this is true. But what they *don't* tell you is that despite the fact that the same kinds of test-tube studies have also conclusively demonstrated that condoms are impenetrable to semen and that spermicides kill all sperm, many unwanted pregnancies occur with the use of condoms and spermicides!

We have known all along that what works in the laboratory does not necessarily work in the bedroom. Dozens of birth control studies, done in many different countries by many reputable scientists, have proved that in actual practice condoms are a poor method of contraception, with a minimum of a 10 percent failure rate for any one year of use! In other words, 1 out of 10 women who regularly and conscientiously use condoms becomes pregnant within a single year (even when it doesn't break).*

The fact is no one has done any scientific studies on how the performance of condoms in test tubes compares with their effectiveness in protecting you from the AIDS virus in real life. Actually there are several good reasons to believe the failure rate of condoms for protecting women against the AIDS virus could be significantly higher than 10 percent. For one, the AIDS virus is much smaller than the relatively gigantic sperm, and so it can probably get

* Scientific References, Group III: Condoms.

into the moist pubic hair and also escape out over the rim during thrusting much more easily. In addition, we know that free virus particles and AIDS-laden cells are present in an infected man's pre-ejaculatory fluid, which he secretes *before he puts on his condom.* Also, please remember that *all* your partner's body fluids and secretions contain AIDS virus if he is a carrier, *not just his semen,* and condoms offer no protection against these other sources of infection. Finally, as Dr. Theresa Crenshaw has pointed out, most women are fertile for only two to four days each month, but are susceptible to AIDS each time they make love to an infected man!

It is most important for you to realize that even though condoms have been widely advertised as providing "safe sex" for women, at this writing not a single study has been published demonstrating that in real life condoms protect women, or men for that matter, against AIDS.

The Food and Drug Administration would never allow any drug or medical device to be released to the public or to be advertised as effective *without a single successful field trial!* Yet the only reputable scientific investigation of the effectiveness of condoms in preventing the heterosexual transmission of AIDS in real life, albeit small, in fact shows an alarmingly high failure rate.

A careful study by Dr. Margaret Fischl and her colleagues at the University of Miami School of Medicine followed 32 heterosexual couples where one partner had AIDS but the other one did not.

Eight of these couples abstained from sex after learning that one partner had AIDS. None of the healthy spouses of these patients became infected, although they continued to live in the same household. Fourteen couples chose to continue to have sex without using condoms. Within eighteen months, 12 (85 percent) of the previously healthy partners had become infected, presumably through heterosexual transmission.

The most troubling finding was the high failure rate of condoms in the 10 couples who had elected to continue their sexual relationship, but always used condoms. When the study was published in the *Journal of the American Medical Association* in February 1987, one of the previously healthy spouses (10 percent) had already become infected within eighteen months! By May 1987 another healthy wife whose husband used condoms regularly had become infected.* A third woman in the condom-using group also seroconverted, but it is not clear if she belonged to the original 10 couples. That represents a 20 or 30 percent failure rate within a two-year period!

. The study clearly shows that there is a high failure rate. But more evidence is needed to permit drawing valid conclusions about how many women will get AIDS if they rely on condoms. The investigators are studying more couples at this time, and so are others, and we will have to wait and see what the real truth about condoms and AIDS is. Meanwhile, though, if you rely on condoms alone, you are playing Russian roulette with your life.

The decision to continue to have sex but to reduce the risks with condoms could be a wise and loving choice for a woman who is already in a relationship with an infected man. However, even the most conservative estimate of a 10 percent failure rate seems to me unacceptable for protecting single women, especially very young women, who should not find it difficult to *eliminate* the risk. They do not have to gamble their lives and the lives of their future babies on condoms.

THERE IS AN IMPORTANT PLACE FOR CONDOMS

I am not "against" the appropriate use of condoms to reduce the risks. But I am very much opposed to exaggerating the protection afforded by condoms and giving women a dangerous false sense of security.

* Personal communication with the authors.

Condoms are probably the single most cost-effective risk-reduction measure for sexually active homosexual men, and also for men and women in countries with limited resources, and in communities where AIDS is widespread among everyone. Their use should not be discouraged in communities that have no other choice because of lack of facilities for comprehensive testing and education programs. But condoms are not a panacea for American women. They are a "quick fix" that can only reduce, not eliminate, the risk of contracting AIDS and should be considered as a second-best line of defense for you. Moreover condoms should be *used only as part of a comprehensive program* that includes education and testing to establish the AIDS status of sexual partners. This has been recommended by such prestigious and responsible public health organizations and professionals as the United States Centers for Disease Control, experts on AIDS at the National Institutes of Health, and the AIDS task force of AASECT (the American Association for Sex Educators, Counselors, and Therapists), among others.* Condoms also make sense for places like certain regions in central Africa where the disease has spread throughout all groups of men, women, and children, making it difficult to identify and avoid sex with infected persons.

But this is not the case here. Condoms are less useful here because the disease is almost entirely confined to two relatively small high-risk groups, who can be easily identified and targeted for preventive efforts.

Condoms are valuable for reducing the risks for anyone, man or woman, who has, for good reasons, chosen to risk possible or even definite exposure to sexual transmission of the AIDS virus.

But for the most part an American woman's first choice should be *eliminating risk by avoiding sex with infected men* and she should rely on condoms only under a few special circumstances.

---

* Scientific References, Group IV, The AIDS Tests, Counseling, and Prevention.

Table 7 *When Condoms Should Be Used*

- By high-risk males who do not want to forgo sex with other high-risk individuals (I.V. drug users with other drug users, male homosexuals with other homosexuals).

- By low-risk males who don't want to forgo sex with high-risk females (men who frequent prostitutes, sailors on leave in African ports, sexually compulsive men).

- As a cost-effective public health measure for men and women who live in countries where AIDS is widespread and evenly distributed and where the educational or medical facilities for comprehensive AIDS testing are not available.

- By women who wish to take a calculated and informed risk with high-risk men, or with men who are known to be infected with AIDS.

- By women who wish to have sex with low-risk men in low-risk circumstances (see Chapter 5) before they are sure about the man's AIDS status.

- *For prevention you do not need condoms if both of you are uninfected or if you are both infected.* *

* There is some concern that repeated exposure may aggravate existing HIV infections.

A woman may have good reason to choose the risk because she loves a man who is a known AIDS carrier or who is already ill with AIDS. If you are in this position and you make an informed choice, condoms are invaluable for reducing the risk of your becoming infected.

I can see where a woman who is married to or in love with a man who has AIDS may decide that she is willing to take a chance in order to continue the sexual closeness that means a great deal to both during the last years of his life.

I had a patient, a woman of forty-five, who had been living for many years with a bisexual man. They had a completely open and caring and mutually supportive relationship. When they learned that he had AIDS, she chose to continue their sexual connection with protection. I supported her in her decision since she understood all the facts, she was not planning to have any more children, and she knew what her priorities were. This couple have been using barrier contraception † conscientiously, and I am keeping my fingers crossed.

† Barrier contraception refers to the use of condoms and diaphragms, which work by physically barring the sperm's entrance into the woman's womb.

You may be so deeply in love with an infected man that making love to him is your first priority and you are willing to gamble. In such circumstances, condoms will stack the odds in your favor, but no one can tell you how much. As long as you know that condoms can't protect you completely, it is your life and sometimes you should listen to your heart.

But a word of warning is in order here. Many people have a self-destructive streak within themselves that will sabotage them when they least expect it.

If you have decided to take the risk in continuing or even starting a sexual relationship with an AIDS carrier or with a man who has AIDS, or with a high-risk man, please face yourself honestly and deeply, and make sure that your motive is a *healthy* love or a decent feeling of compassion. AIDS is nothing to play around with. Be sure you are not gambling your life and future because of some neurotic self-destructiveness or a false sense of guilt.

It is not your fault that he has AIDS. Do not feel guilty that you are okay. Keep it that way. If he cares for you he would not want you to commit suttee. We are many years away from that ancient Indian custom which demanded a widow die with her husband by throwing herself to burn alive on his funeral pyre.

DON'T BECOME A VICTIM OF FEAR

AIDS can be used self-destructively by women to avoid love, sex, and romance. Some women who are unconsciously afraid of love and sex and who have deeply buried conflicts about enjoying a successful romantic relationship become obsessed with the Fear of AIDS, which Dr. Harold Lief* has called FAIDS. These fears are not realistic but are being used by these women to sabotage their chances for romantic happiness.

* Dr. Harold Lief is the director of the Family Council in Philadelphia.

If you find that you are avoiding socializing with men because you are afraid of AIDS, or if you are turning off dates with your obsessions about AIDS, look yourself in the mirror. Be honest; do you have a long history of obsessions? Have you been obsessed first with this thing and then with that all your life? Maybe you have an obsessive personality and FAIDS is just your latest obsession. Also ask yourself honestly, do you find yourself anxious and uncomfortable and not at your best around men? Do you have a poor track record in the romantic relationship department? Does it never seem to work out for you? Do you always end up being rejected? Do you always manage to pick the "wrong" man? Do you lose interest in men who are good to you?

If the answer to any of these questions is yes, you need a bit of insight into your deeper neurotic conflicts about sex or about your irrational fear of romantic success. AIDS may just be your latest instrument of self-torture, and I would venture that if the AIDS crisis did not exist you would be beating yourself up with something else.

AIDS is dangerous, of course. That is what this book is all about. However, if you use your head and follow the rules, there is no reason why you can't have a wonderful, romantic, sexy relationship with a man and still remain safe.

HOW TO USE CONDOMS

If you are going to use condoms you might as well make sure your partner uses them properly, for maximum risk reduction. But remember, *you can get AIDS even if the condom does not break!*

The process could surely take all the romance and spontaneity out of sex. But if you want to have intercourse with a man whose AIDS status you do not know, better be as safe as you can be.

Table 8 *How to Use Condoms*

1. Use only latex condoms. Lambskin and other natural membranes feel nicer but are not of proven laboratory effectiveness against the AIDS virus.

2. Do not use saliva as a lubricant. Saliva of an infected person contains the AIDS virus.

3. Do not use oily lubricants. This might dissolve some condoms.

4. He should put some KY lubricant on the tip of his penis.

5. Make sure he leaves a small space free of air, near the tip of his penis, so that when he ejaculates the condom does not break.

6. Make sure he uses a new condom when he has sex with you. Condoms should never be reused, because it is difficult to sterilize them. (If you want to be certain, bring your own.)

7. Use a spermicide that contains nonoxynol-9. This has been shown to inactivate the AIDS virus and slow down infected lymphocytes in *laboratory* experiments. I don't know if it helps, but it wouldn't hurt.

8. Some authorities are now recommending "double" barrier protection, meaning that you use a diaphragm with contraceptive jelly, in addition to his wearing a condom.

9. Inspect the condom for holes and defects before he uses it.

10. Ask him to put the condom on before you have intercourse and as soon as he has an erection as you begin foreplay, because his pre-ejaculatory fluid may be infected, as may your vaginal lubrication.

11. Immediately after he ejaculates, you must both go to the bathroom and wash up. If you are going to snuggle together afterwards, he must remove the condom and wash his penis and pubic area with soap and water and either rubbing alcohol or dilute solutions of lysol.

12. Some men cannot function with a condom, especially as they age. Don't insist, he can't help it. Stick to dry sex.

AIDS TESTING

Testing for AIDS, together with accurate information about safe sex, is the best protection women and adolescents have against AIDS. AIDS testing is the only way to check out if your partner or you have AIDS for sure, and this is the only way you can virtually *eliminate* the risks of your contracting AIDS from your lover or husband.

But nothing has created more political heat and controversy and confusion than AIDS testing, and you might be hearing deceptive and frightening information.

Despite the misinformation or lies you may have been told, AIDS tests are excellent. Actually, they are among the most valid, accurate, and reliable medical tests that are used today.*

Two types of tests are used in combination to determine a person's AIDS status.

The first test that is taken is a screening test called *ELISA* (Enzyme-Linked Immunosorbent Assay), which detects antibodies for the AIDS virus in your blood serum with extreme accuracy. If the results are positive, the test is repeated to make sure there was no laboratory error. This is the usual procedure doctors use with any significantly abnormal lab result.†

If the ELISA AIDS antibody screening test is again positive on retesting, it is always followed by a much more complicated and expensive confirmatory test, the *Western blot test*. This is done to make sure that the antibody that has been picked up by the screening test is really and truly an AIDS antibody, and not some other kind of similar but non-AIDS antibody.

Most virus diseases are diagnosed by finding antibodies to them in the person's bloodstream. The virus itself is rarely actually isolated except in investigative studies or by specialized laboratories because virus particles are difficult to find, and they must be grown in tissue culture cells, which is difficult, tedious, and very labor-intensive.

---

* Scientific References, Group IV: The AIDS Tests, Counseling, and Prevention.
† For example, if I am evaluating a patient with an erection problem, I often want to make sure that he does not have poor penile circulation, early diabetes, or a silent hormone deficiency which can also cause impotence. So I order some tests, and if these indicate that he has an abnormality, following accepted medical procedure I always repeat the test, and sometimes include more reliable diagnostic procedures, before I tell the patient that there is something wrong with him I prescribe hormone replacement or suggest insulin treatment.

The validity of antibody tests for AIDS has been thoroughly checked by scientists who actually did go to the considerable trouble of isolating the HIV virus from patients who are positive on the tests, and the AIDS virus has been grown in the laboratory. These studies have conclusively proved that the tests are highly reliable.

The ELISA screening test for AIDS is so finely tuned for detecting the presence of AIDS antibodies that practically no one with antibodies slips through the "screen." However, any test that is very sensitive will sometimes give "false positive" results. This means that the test will come out positive for AIDS antibodies even though the person does not have AIDS. For example, a person might get false positive readings if he has *similar* antibodies in his blood for a disease such as malaria.

Therefore, if both screening ELISA tests come out positive, they are always followed by a confirmatory Western blot test before the diagnosis of AIDS infection is made, or before the patient is told that he or she has been infected with the AIDS virus.

When *both tests are used together* the chances are close to 100 percent that a person who is positive in both tests has really been infected by the AIDS virus.

It is much easier to tell if a person does *not* have the AIDS virus, because the ELISA screening test has practically no "false negatives." In other words, it almost never falsely indicates that a person with AIDS is free of infection. That is of course exactly what you want to know about your prospective partner before you go to bed with him.

THE WINDOW

But there is a "window" of time before the antibody shows up in an infected person's bloodstream. This is a potential pitfall. You must protect yourself against the danger of "falling through the window," but this is really very simple, if you understand the true facts. Do *not* let anyone undermine your confidence in AIDS testing by exaggerating the perils of the *antibody window*.

A person is infected and infectious to you as soon as the virus enters the cells of his body. But it takes the immune system a little time before it can manufacture AIDS antibodies. The period between infection and before the antibodies can be detected in the blood is called "the window." The great majority of people produce antibodies within two weeks, and certainly by the sixth week after they have been infected over 90 percent of infected persons are *seropositive*. However, for a few people this takes as long as six months, by which time over 99% show up positive.*

Therefore, a person should wait six weeks after he or she has been exposed before having a screening test, and should certainly abstain from sexual intercourse (with or without condoms) during this time. If the test is negative, there is a very good chance that the person is okay, but he should take it again six months later, if you have any doubts.

If it already has been six months since you were exposed, you only need to be tested once, because the window has already passed for the great majority of people.

A negative test result shows that you and/or your partner had no antibodies in your bloodstream when you took the test. But your AIDS status is still not absolutely certain if the exposure took place very recently. This is a matter of judgment. If the chances that you were exposed are low and your test is negative, you are most probably okay. But if the chances of exposure are considerable, I would suggest that the person wait and see until he or she is retested later.

For example, if he had a blood transfusion three months *ago* and he tests negative, there is probably less than one chance in ten million (that's 0.00001 percent) that he is infected, and I personally would accept that risk.

* In *extremely rare* cases seroconversion may take as long as 14 months.

Or if he once slept with a prostitute from a low-risk area (see Figure 4 in Chapter 4) four months ago and the test does not show AIDS antibodies, I would not worry.

But if he had a homosexual encounter three months ago, or went to a "shooting gallery," I would certainly not feel secure if he tests out okay on the first test. I would feel much better. But I would wait for his second test results three months later before I got into wet sex with him. During this time, I would absolutely restrict myself to the "ultrasafe," or "dry," sexual practices described in Chapter 5.

If you and your partner still have no antibodies six months after exposure, there is a 99.9 percent chance that neither he nor you is infected. So if he has passed the test six months after he has been exposed, and you are sure that he is not sleeping with anyone else or shooting drugs, you can make love to him again any way that you like and you can throw away those annoying condoms, diaphragms, and smelly jellies, and disinfectants.

Should your AIDS test come out positive, you have been *infected*. This is bad news and means that the virus has actually entered your body. This does not mean that you have AIDS or are necessarily going to get AIDS. It does mean however that you have an HIV infection, and according to what we currently know, there is a 30 percent to 50 percent chance that you will develop AIDS within seven years. There is some evidence that women seem to be more susceptible to AIDS and die more rapidly once they develop the disease. But the most important thing for you to remember, from an ethical point of view, is that you can transmit the disease to others through blood or sex, and to your baby during pregnancy or through breast-feeding, from now on.

I had hoped to list some reliable AIDS resources here, but the ones I checked were dispensing outdated and inappropriate information for women. Therefore I cannot recommend any particular resource at this time out of concern that I may be giving you poor advice.

Table 9   *When You and Your Partner Should Be Tested*

1. *Six weeks after any possible exposure.*

   a. *Men*

   (1) a "wet" homosexual encounter (i.e., anal or oral sex, with or without condoms),
   (2) sharing a hypodermic needle,
   (3) a "wet" sexual encounter with a "high-risk" woman, including prostitutes, promiscuous women, especially those from high-risk areas, travelers to places where there is a high incidence of HIV infection, or a stranger, or a known AIDS carrier (with or without condoms),
   (4) a blood transfusion.

   b. *Women*

   (1) a "wet" sexual encounter with a bisexual man (with or without condoms),
   (2) sharing a hypodermic needle,
   (3) a "wet" sexual encounter with an I.V. drug user, a stranger, especially one who lives in or travels to high-risk areas, or a known AIDS carrier (with or without a condom),
   (4) a blood transfusion.

If the ELISA test is negative six weeks after exposure, the chances that you are infected are less than 10%.

2. *Six months after exposure you should be retested, just in case the first test was taken during the antibody "window."*

If you are still negative six months later, the chances of your being infected are almost zero.

Negative results on the tests mean you are okay. But positive test results on the ELISA *do not* mean you have AIDS because this sensitive test sometimes gives *false positive* results. You must be retested, and if still positive, a confirmatory *Western blot* test should be done. There is a 99.9% chance that a person who tests positive for HIV antibodies on both tests is infected.

ADOLESCENT GIRLS (AND BOYS)

Dr. Karen Hein, a pediatric AIDS specialist, recently voiced the fears of many experts in a paper which appeared in the May 1987 issue of the *New York State Journal of Medicine*. "Adolescents coming into contact with infected men form the basis of substantial risk which places them directly in the path of the oncoming epidemic." I am most especially concerned that we are not doing enough about the AIDS disaster that is about to impact on young girls in our high schools and our junior high schools.

People really do not appreciate how early kids start experimenting with drugs and sex today. It is not unusual for inner-city ghetto kids to start using I.V. drugs and to become sexually active by the age of ten or eleven. In middle-class public schools and in some of the more liberal upper-class private schools in urban areas, youngsters do not use I.V. drugs so much, but they are also becoming sexually active very early, by the age of twelve or fourteen.

Infectious disease experts have expressed concern that many adolescent boys have become infected with AIDS through homosexual contact and drug addiction. Disadvantaged youngsters from the poorer sections of our large cities are especially at risk. Some are homosexual themselves, while others have been abused by homosexuals or tempted by the "easy" money they can earn for a few minutes of sex. Other boys have become AIDS carriers by sharing needles with their older brothers, pushers, and "pals." A small minority of boys have become infected from sexual contact with infected prostitutes and an even smaller number from drug-using girls in their own peer groups.

Most of these boys do not have the slightest idea that they are infected, and neither do the girls, because AIDS testing is not encouraged or even available in most schools. And since AIDS testing and contact tracing in the schools is strongly opposed by "right to privacy" advocates, I am afraid this is not likely to happen in time to save a lot of young lives. The kids are also being misled by the "use condoms for safe sex" campaigns and therefore do not know the truth about risks. Between these destructive public health policies and peer pressure for early sexual activity our adolescents are facing a real catastrophe.

AIDS AND PREGNANCY

What must you do to preserve your ability to give birth to healthy babies?

Clearly, the best way to prevent exposing and infecting your future children to AIDS while you are carrying them is to avoid exposure and infection yourself. This is an absolute guarantee against giving birth to babies with AIDS.

Exactly how many babies of seropositive mothers will be infected with AIDS through intrauterine transmission is not known for certain at this time, but it looks very grim. One excellent study found that 35 percent of first children of seropositive mothers are born infected, and the figure rose to 65 percent of their subsequent babies. But other investigations now under way here and abroad suggest that the fetal infection rate will probably turn out to be about 50 percent and, sadly, the majority of these children are expected to die.

You have to be careful, but at this point in time there is no need to panic because the great majority of American women today are not yet infected. If you are planning to have a baby the chances that you are infected, in order of increasing risks, is as follows:

1. If you and your husband are not in a high-risk group, and especially if you have been monogamous, the chances are so overwhelmingly good that you have not been infected that you can simply forget about worrying. I would say, go ahead and plan your family.

2. If you have had a blood transfusion between 1978, when the virus first began to contaminate our blood supply and 1984, when the blood banks were able to test the blood, the risk is still very small. If you have had a transfusion after 1984, the chances that you have been infected are

even smaller, estimated to be only one in 250,000 (0.0025 percent).* But why not get tested and be sure?

3. If you have had some casual sexual encounters during the past eight years, especially if you do not live in a high-risk area (see Figure 4 in Chapter 4), you are still most probably not infected. Each year, however, there are more heterosexually active infected males, so the risks if you had an affair in 1986 are a bit higher than they were in 1979, but the odds are still overwhelmingly against your lover's having been a carrier of the AIDS virus, especially if you are white and middle-class. Unless you have had many high-risk partners, you're probably still okay. But if it is possible that even one of your partners was infected, check it out. Get tested before you get pregnant.

4. The only women who need to be really concerned about giving birth to a baby with AIDS are I.V. drug users and the partners of I.V. drug users, hemophiliacs, and bisexuals. Black and Hispanic women are especially vulnerable. If you are in one of these situations, you are definitely at risk. You should have yourself tested before you have a baby.

Because the risk of your baby's becoming infected during pregnancy is so high, many health authorities have recommended that premarital testing be mandatory or at least encouraged, and some obstetricians are recommending that all high-risk women † be tested during pregnancy.

But in most cases it will be up to *you* to find out if you are a carrier. If your community does not require, and/or your doctor doesn't encourage, premarital or prenatal AIDS testing, and if there is the slightest doubt in your mind that you or your fiancé or husband have been exposed, you and he should both be tested before you get married and/or *before you try to become* pregnant.

The few unfortunate women who are already infected,

---

* Scientific References, Group VII: Transmission of AIDS by Infected Blood.
† Prostitutes, I.V. drug users, women with a sexual history of exposure to multiple partners, and women whose partners are high-risk males.

and those who are married to infected men, have a difficult personal decision to make if they want to start a family or if the pregnancy is already under way.

You and your husband have several choices, all of them difficult. You may require counseling to help you. If pregnant, you will have to decide whether to take the chance that the baby might be okay, or to have an abortion. If you were planning to have a family, you have to choose whether to take the chance, or try to adopt, or to accept being childless. If your husband is infected but you are not, you might want to have a baby by artificial insemination from a healthy donor. You also have to consider the baby's future in light of the sad fact that the odds that the infected parent will be ill, disabled, or dead within 7 years may be as high as 50 percent.

If you and/or your husband are infected, you are in a position similar to that of couples who find one or both have a genetic defect. Genetic counseling can be very helpful in these cases, and a skilled professional will give you the facts as well as the emotional support you need.

The risk of neonatal infection seems to go up with each pregnancy, and the health of infected women tends to deteriorate during pregnancy. For both these reasons many physicians are now recommending that women who have HIV infections never have children, and are advising those who are already pregnant to terminate their pregnancy and not to get pregnant again. On the other hand, the Roman Catholic Church and the Orthodox Jewish rabbinate are absolutely against this.

Again, it is your life, and your baby, and ultimately *you* must decide for yourself, together with your husband.

BLOOD: REDUCING THE RISKS

Prior to 1986, contact with infected blood was the most common route of transmission of AIDS to women in this country. (Now it is sex.)

Here is how you can avoid or reduce the risks of getting AIDS through infected blood:

1. Do not use *intravenous drugs.* Drug abuse is self-destructive for many reasons which are self-evident. If you are addicted you know that you need help, and that you should enroll in a drug rehabilitation program. But if you can't kick the habit right now, at least use new needles, or wash the needles with a bleach solution before you use them, and *do not share your needles with anyone!**

2. Avoid contact with *contaminated blood.* Hospital cleaning personnel, laboratory technicians, nurse's aides, dental technicians, nurses, dentists, and doctors (especially surgeons and pathologists) are frequently in contact with blood from infected patients. This is potentially dangerous because the blood contains both free HIV virus and infected cells. We do not yet know what the exact level of danger for health workers caring for AIDS-infected patients is, but I am afraid that it might turn out to be higher than we were led to believe.†

Health personnel have now been advised to wear rubber gloves and masks while caring for AIDS patients and carriers, and cautioned to be extremely careful to avoid injuries related to caring for the ill. It would be helpful if patients undergoing surgical procedures could be tested for AIDS and identified, but there is great political opposition to this.

* Only drugs which are injected by hypodermic needle are implicated in the transmission of AIDS. These are mostly narcotics, including heroin, morphine and Demerol. Those which are taken by mouth or inhaled, including alcohol, "uppers," "downers," marijuana, and cocaine, do not spread the AIDS virus but are destructive for other reasons.

† On May 20, 1987, the CDC, which along with the World Health Organization of the United Nations had until then taken the position that health personnel caring for patients with AIDS were "in no danger," issued a report that three female nurses, who worked at different hospitals, became infected when they were splashed by the blood of AIDS patients or carriers. On June 4, 1987, investigators who tested dentists practicing in New York City found that one dentist had already become infected, apparently from fixing the teeth of a "healthy" carrier. Recently two scientists working on laboratory studies of HIV seroconverted.

In the meantime, healthcare workers have rights too! And if you are in the medical field you could exercise your right to have the AIDS status of patients you are caring for be determined, so that you can take the same precautions that are standard procedure for patients with other diseases transmitted through infected body fluids, such as hepatitis B.

3. Avoid potentially contaminated blood products. Receiving a transfusion of AIDS-infected blood is exceedingly dangerous, and a high proportion of recipients of infected blood have now been infected. For example, up to 80 percent of hemophiliacs in some areas of the country are now infected because they received contaminated blood products. *

The story of blood-transmitted AIDS should have taught us a lesson, but it didn't.

Early on it was noticed that in San Francisco and other high-risk areas, cases of AIDS were being reported in patients who had received blood transfusions. It was immediately understood that blood donated by infected persons, mainly homosexuals, was responsible for this disaster. The AIDS screening tests had not yet been developed, but it was against the Red Cross Blood Program policy to exclude blood donors on the basis of sexual orientation, with the result that many transfusion recipients were killed by AIDS-contaminated blood. †

To date, 404 male and 202 female transfusion recipients have contracted AIDS, ‡ and since compulsory contact tracing is not done in many parts of the country, no one knows how many were infected who are not ill yet. Since the ratio of symptomatic to asymptomatic patients is thought to be 100 to 1 (see Figure 2), even though some infected blood recipients have undoubtedly died of other causes, it may be estimated that 30,000 to 50,000 men,

---

* Hemophiliacs rely on blood products made from a fraction of the blood of as many as 75,000 individuals.
† Scientific References, Group VII: Transmission of AIDS by Infected Blood.
‡ For other dangerous communicable diseases, contact tracing and notification is required by law in many states. It is sheer lunacy to exempt AIDS!

women, and children have been infected through contaminated blood and are now "healthy" AIDS carriers. It is tragic that public health officials in many communities failed to find out who the carriers were so that they could be notified and could in turn protect their sexual partners.

When the news got out, the country's blood supply program, which is crucial to our medical care system, became a shambles; it was so bad that some foreign countries would not allow U.S. blood products to cross their borders!

Fortunately, the problem was largely solved when the AIDS tests were perfected in 1985. Since that time all donated blood has been tested and screened for additional safety, and the blood products that hemophiliacs require are now treated with heat, which kills the AIDS virus.

But hospitals and blood banks still do not test donors. However, it is now the Red Cross's policy to attempt to *discourage* high-risk individuals from donating blood. Unfortunately when a donor's AIDS antibody test indicates that he is infected, the individual is counseled to use "safe" sexual practices, i.e., condoms. But the AIDS carriers, 93 percent of whom are male, are *not told* to desist from having sex with uninfected partners.

Because such high-risk individuals are not entirely excluded, a very tiny fraction of contaminated blood, probably about one in 250,000 transfusions,* is still slipping through the testing screen into our blood supply because if the blood of an infected person is tested during the earliest stage of infection known as the "antibody window," the virus in the blood will not show up on the test.

So please, if you are going to have an elective operation, arrange to donate your own blood ahead of time if this is medically feasible, and let your doctor have it stored for you so he or she can use it in case you need a transfusion. Some surgeons and hospitals will object to your request for an *autologous transfusion* † because this creates additional

---

* See Appendix H.
† Being transfused with your own blood is called an "autologous" blood transfusion. This is highly recommended by many responsible and caring obstetricians and surgeons.

work for them. But you should stand up for your rights. What is a bit of bother compared to even a small reduction in the risk of getting AIDS!

Even if you are pregnant, and especially if you are going to have your baby by cesarean delivery, which might necessitate a transfusion, you can give your own blood well before the due date and have your doctors store it just in case.

If you are scheduled to have an operation that could involve substantial blood loss, such as a hysterectomy or a coronary artery bypass, and you cannot give your own blood for medical reasons, the next best thing to do is find a friend or a relative from a low-risk group who has the right type of blood, and ask him or her to be tested and to donate blood earmarked for you.

If it turns out that you did not need a transfusion after all, someone else will benefit from the uncontaminated blood.

Please note: You *can not* get AIDS by *giving* blood, only by *receiving* contaminated blood! And donating blood is an excellent way of getting tested for free if you have any doubts about your AIDS status. But *please*, do not do this for 6 months after your last exposure!

5

Great Safe Sex
in the
Age of AIDS

Although there are highly unusual circumstances, like that of the unfortunate nurses who were infected by blood from patients with AIDS, *sex with an infected man is essentially the only route of infection you need to worry about*. But there are great differences in the degrees of risk involved in various sexual practices and circumstances. All other things being equal, even assuming that your partner has AIDS, the danger to you ranges from zero to 100 percent, depending on what you do in bed.

At this writing, most so-called "AIDS resources" and the how-to-avoid-AIDS books are giving you yesterday's information and it would not be surprising if you are confused. But keep the bottom line in mind: *"Wet sex" is dangerous but "dry sex" is safe*.

By this I mean that all sexual experiences that entail the exchange of any body fluids, not only semen, or contact between your moist surfaces and his, can transmit the AIDS virus and so are *unsafe*, if he should turn out to be infected. The details of how the AIDS virus can invade you through wet parts of your body was explained in Chapter 4.

Therefore, remember:

1. *Vaginal intercourse* is not safe if he is or could be infected (with or without condoms).
2. *Anal intercourse* is not safe if he is or could be infected (with or without condoms).
3. *Oral sex* is not safe,* in either direction, if he is or could be infected. (The AIDS virus can enter your body if he stimulates your genitalia with his mouth, and also if you stimulate his penis orally *even if he does not ejaculate into your mouth.*)
4. *Kissing* the person you love is so pleasurable and such an important expression of intimacy, that it really bothers me that I cannot tell you in all good conscience that wet, or deep, kissing is okay. But the risks entailed in wet kissing are not known. AIDS virus has been found in the saliva of some infected individuals, but since most couples who have intercourse also exchange kisses, the role of kissing in the sexual transmission of AIDS remains unclear.

Incidentally, in case you feel guilty about saying no to wet sex, remember, all these sexual acts are also potentially dangerous for men if *you* are infected.

But there is every reason to believe that if you limit yourself to *dry sex*, and make sure that your partner's fluids do not mingle with your fluids or touch the wet parts of your mouth or genitalia or your nipples, you will be *safe*, even if it should turn out that your partner is an AIDS carrier, because, to quote Dr. A. Fauci, the head of the NIH (National Institutes of Health) AIDS program, "there is

* The heterosexual transmission of AIDS virus through oral sex has not been proved for certain, because it is difficult, if not impossible, to study infected persons who engage only in fellatio or cunnilingus and no other form of sex.

zero evidence" that the virus can enter your body through casual (dry) contact. Again, as far as we know today, HIV cannot infect you in any way except through the moist parts of your body, or by getting directly into your blood.

Let me explain what I mean by "dry sex."

Our sexual organs are directly connected to the pleasure centers of the brain, and many kinds of sexual stimulation, even just thinking of sex, flirting, kissing, and foreplay, all of which are usually merely preliminary to the actual act of intercourse, are also highly pleasurable to us. This fortunate biological arrangement makes it possible for you and your partner to enjoy a number of highly erotic and sensuous experiences together which do not entail sexual intercourse, oral sex, anal sex, or any other form of dangerous "wet" sex which involves the mingling of body fluids, or contact of body fluids with moist mucous membranes.

I am speaking here solely about medical safety, and not about morality or personal preference. So please do not take the following descriptions of safe or "ultralow-risk" sexual practices as suggestions or recommendations. I just want you to know that they are, according to the best scientific information available to date, safe from the standpoint of catching AIDS. If you have any moral, personal, or emotional objections to or reservations about fantasy or masturbation or any of the other safe or safer erotic activities described below, you should not do them!

But many perfectly nice, decent people have no qualms about touching each other's bodies, mutual masturbation, or sharing sexually arousing fantasies and films, which are all safe sexual practices. If both partners are comfortable with these forms of sexual stimulation and find them arousing and fulfilling, you can share deeply gratifying sexual experiences with your man without taking chances with your life.

But many people avoid any form of sex except straight sexual intercourse because they mistakenly think everything else is sick or childish or immoral. That is not true from a medical or scientific point of view. It is just as normal *not* to like and to avoid any or all of these as it is to enjoy them, and it just so happens that fantasy and manual genital stimulation are the keys to *great safe sex*.

The freedom to enjoy these safe forms of sexual expression is especially valuable for women who do not want to, or for some reasons cannot, choose monogamy. Dry sex can also be an excellent interim experience for couples who are still deciding whether to commit themselves permanently to a relationship.

MONOGAMY

The risks of infection become greater with each additional partner. If you can enjoy sex within a committed monogamous relationship you are much better off. But some people lack the capacity for melding sexual arousal with emotional closeness. They are turned on by anonymous sex with strangers and they become sexually blocked when a relationship becomes emotionally too close or committed for them. If your man has this problem, he is risky for you! These people suffer from "emotional claustrophobia" when a relationship exceeds their "intimacy comfort zone," and they feel trapped and frustrated if they are not free to have sex with others.

Men are more likely to have a low tolerance for monogamy, and to suffer from inhibited sexual desire in sexually exclusive relationships. However, we are now beginning to see some women who also have problems with commitment and/or intimacy. These unfortunate individuals are turned off sexually by emotional closeness and end up with lonely lives. Happily they are a relatively small group. Most women, and many men also, find that sex with an intimate partner, with someone to whom one is emotionally close, and with whom one feels a total mutual acceptance, and within a relationship where no one needs to posture or put on an act, is the ultimate sexual experience.

That is not to say that a healthy person can't also enjoy a lovely sensuous interlude with an attractive stranger. Many normal men and women can and do. But this has become dangerous in the age of AIDS.

It is true that the majority of couples who have been together for a long time lose some of the intense erotic desire for each other which is typical of the beginning of a new relationship (although for a small number of lucky people the spouse remains their sexual fantasy forever). Many couples who have been in long-term relationships still enjoy sex together and have no problems functioning, but the initial sexual "heat" tends to diminish over the years. In good marriages the intense passion is replaced by a sense of closeness and comfort in the bedroom.

Some couples who have been together for a long time complain that sex gets boring and some even develop a dysfunction or a pattern of sexual avoidance, which they attribute to the long duration of the relationship. But these kinds of complaints are never just due to "boredom." Sexual difficulties of this sort are a sign of hidden marital problems and anger between the partners, and *not* a natural outcome of long-lasting monogamy.* The sex therapy methods that can often help to revive the sex lives of such couples are discussed later on, because some of these techniques could make your sexual relationship with your partner more exciting while you remain safe. The same sexual fantasy and "dry" stimulation techniques which help patients overcome their sexual problems could help you have high-quality safe sex with partners whose AIDS status you are not sure of.

INTIMACY

Whether or not you are in a sexually exclusive relationship, intimacy improves all connections between two people,

* Scientific References, Group VIII: Sex Therapy and Sexology.

and certainly makes every sexual encounter more enjoyable and comfortable. Intimacy means that you openly share your genuine feelings with your partner in a close and caring way. This open communication about what each of you likes and dislikes sexually, and what you each need, and what makes you feel vulnerable is an important ingredient of all good sexual relationships.

It takes some time to get to know your partner, to learn if you can trust each other, and to find out whether he has been exposed to AIDS or whether he is safe. This waiting period is a perfect opportunity for you to establish an intimate relationship. You are not rushing to have sex, you are just learning to be together. You are finding out about each other's most personal erotic desires and sensitivities while you are free of sexual performance pressures and sexual anxieties.

Sex therapists often deliberately ask couples to abstain from sexual intercourse during the initial stages of treatment to free them from their self-made pressure to perform and from their obsession with "proving" their sexual prowess to their partners. During this time they learn to be intimate, to make close emotional contact with each other, to communicate their feelings to each other. A period of abstinence from intercourse gives couples the chance to learn what it takes to make each other comfortable and sexually satisfied.

At a later phase of therapy we often prescribe special "homework" assignments that get couples used to touching and caressing each other's bodies in a nonpressured and sensitive way, in order to heighten their capacity for sensual pleasure and to diminish their sexual fears and guilts — while they are still free from the pressure to perform sexual intercourse. These therapeutic techniques were called by their inventors, Masters and Johnson, "sensate focus exercises." *

Sex therapists now use numerous variations of such sen-

* Scientific References, Group VIII: Sex Therapy and Sexology.

suous and erotic "pre-intercourse" experiences to help anxious and inexperienced couples learn to relax in bed, and to "desensitize" their sexual anxieties and to get rid of their performance panics.

For example, we might suggest that couples take "intimate showers" together. They soap and wash each other gently and slowly and then they dry and powder each other, without proceeding to intercourse, just for the fun of it, and just to get used to being physical with each other. This provides patients the opportunity, often for the first time in their lives, to look at the body and genitalia, to gently touch, to play with a member of the opposite sex in a nonpressured relaxed atmosphere.

DRY SEX

These therapeutic "sensate focus" techniques and "intimacy exercises" are relevant to our discussion of dry sex because body caressing happens to be a form of dry sex considered entirely safe from the standpoint of transmitting AIDS. These games are not to everyone's taste, but if the idea of nude showers and exploring each other's bodies does not appeal to you and your partner, you could develop your own versions of sensate focus and share physical pleasures together safely, while you are getting to know each other, or while you are deciding on commitment, or while you are waiting to feel safe with him.

But a word of caution. Being alone together nude and touching each other might be very arousing to your partner and to you too, and he may press you for "wet" sex: sexual intercourse or oral sex, even though you had both agreed and made a "deal" to abstain. Be prepared for his urging you to do this. He is only human, but nicely and absolutely refuse.

DRY KISSING
Kissing your partner with your mouth closed on the lips or body (but *not* the genitals or nipples) is safe, and can be extremely enjoyable.

Sadly, I cannot reassure you that exchanging saliva with an infected partner is safe. Therefore, even though it might be difficult to abstain from deep, or wet, kissing as you become more intimate with your man, until we know more, I would advise against it.*

DRY BODY CONTACT

Another safe dry sexual practice which men particularly enjoy is for the two of you to rhythmically rub against each other's bodies and genitalia for arousal and/or orgasm while you both have your clothes on. A date's thrusting his penis against you was a very popular sexual practice in my generation, when "nice girls" did not "go all the way." This was called "dry humping," and is *ultrasafe*.

If you are careful you can press together in the nude. But, again watch out! This can be very exciting! Do not let yourself be tempted to go beyond the bounds of safety!

If he rubs his penis against your side or buttock, but *not near your anus or external genitals (vulva)*, you are still pretty safe, especially if he wears a condom. It is also okay if he rubs himself against your belly or thigh. But do not let him come anywhere *near* your pubic hair or genitalia. Remember, the moist skin of your anus and genitalia and your nipples are potential entrance ports for the AIDS virus. That whole area is moist when you are excited, and the AIDS bugs can "swim" right into your body that way. You must wash immediately and disinfect the places where his semen wet you.

With the same precaution, you can rub your clitoris against the dry skin of his arm or his thigh to arouse yourself and/or to stimulate yourself to orgasm.

You will definitely be safer if he wears a condom, but even then, only let him ejaculate on the dry parts of your body.

PARALLEL ORGASM

You may choose to go further and explore some more intense sexual experiences that are a little more hazardous,

* Scientific References, Group VI: Heterosexual Transmission of AIDS.

but can still be considered "ultralow risk," if you are very careful. Parallel orgasm has very low risk if you do not get wet. Do not allow your partner's potentially infectious secretions to touch your vulnerable moist skin, or mucous membranes, or get into any nicks or abrasions or sores you may have on your "dry" skin.

Simultaneously masturbating yourselves in each other's presence, manually or with a vibrator, is medically safe as long as you do not get semen on any body openings, specifically on the moist mucous membranes that cover your genitalia and the openings of your nipples. This is also safe for him, provided he does not get any of your genital lubrication on the urethral opening of his penis or, if he is uncircumcised, on the moist tip of the penis underneath his foreskin.

Stimulating yourselves to orgasms, manually or with a vibrator, even if you are not touching each other, can be extremely exciting and gratifying for many couples. By observing each other's arousal and climax, you are sharing a very private experience with each other. You are allowing yourselves to be vulnerable with each other. Apart from being safe from the standpoint of eliminating any risks of becoming infected with AIDS, when two people let their guard down and see that they will not get hurt, it makes them feel more loving and close to each other.

Parallel masturbation can be even more exciting if you combine the physical stimulation of your genitalia with your and/or his favorite fantasy.

Stimulating *each other* to orgasm can also be considered very low risk as long as you do not get his pre-ejaculatory secretions or his semen on any of your body openings, or on your nipples, or on your hand if you have open hangnail sores, scratches, or wounds. If you are wearing a Band-Aid on one of your hands use the other one.

The rule is "keep it dry." If you should "wet" each other, you must get up at once and wash any part of your body that has been in contact with the potentially infected fluid. Scrub with soap and water in addition to disinfecting the area with undiluted rubbing alcohol or a dilute solution of Lysol.* This is important. It is not so dangerous if his semen gets on your hands, especially if it gets on the *thick skin* of the palms of your hands which is less easily broken and more protective than the *thin skin* on the other parts of the body. But if you do not wash it off it will stay on your hands, and if you bite your nails, or eat something with your fingers a few hours later, some virus might have survived and you could become infected.

Again, remember you may be able to get infected if virus-laden fluid gets into cuts, scratches, or other little wounds and pimples on your skin; even pierced ears may give the virus access to your body! †

FRICTION AND FANTASY

There are two essential ingredients for good sex: friction and fantasy.

Friction is really a tricky way of saying that both the male sexual reflexes (erection and ejaculation), and the female sexual reflexes (vaginal lubrication and orgasm) are triggered by *rhythmic physical stimulation of the genitalia.*

Fantasy is a catchword for *psychic stimulation*, which is also needed, along with physical stimulation, for men and women to function physically and to enjoy the experience. Young men can often attain an erection by either physical or psychological stimulation alone. Older men usually need a combination of psychic *and* physical stimulation to attain or to maintain an erection. And women of all ages can become aroused and lubricated from either physical

---

* Do *not* put rubbing alcohol, Lysol, or any other strong disenfectant on your genitalia, and *never* douche your vagina with those liquids, or you will get a nasty inflammation. Do not let any potentially infected secretions get there in the first place!

† Although this possibility *is extremely remote*, the CDC (Centers for Disease Control) speculated that one nurse might have been infected with AIDS virus when infected blood splashed on her pierced ear.

caresses or from psychological stimulation alone. But *simultaneous* psychic *and* physical stimulation are generally needed for women and for men to reach a climax.

Women receive the physical stimulation they need for arousal by foreplay, when the partner caresses and kisses their body and the erotic zones of the lips and the nipples and the genital area. Women usually reach orgasm by direct manual or oral stimulation of the clitoris, or by the indirect clitoral stimulation which is provided by their partner's rhythmic thrusting during intercourse. Vaginal stimulation by the partner's penis and/or fingers is also very pleasurable, and this alone brings some women (about 25 percent) to orgasm.

Men are also aroused by foreplay, and they reach orgasm and ejaculation when their penis is rhythmically stimulated manually, orally, or by thrusting into their partner's vagina.

The mental image of your lover and your awareness of the exciting things you are doing together supplies the essential *psychological component*. It is also very common to heighten your sexual arousal by mentally conjuring up sexual fantasies, erotic images, and romantic memories, and by using explicit erotic literature, pictures, and films.

Psychic sexual stimulation, or fantasy, plays such an important role in all good sex that it has been said that "the brain is the most important sexual organ in the body."

Unless you happen to *be* his sexual fantasy, you cannot be a really great sexual partner unless you understand what excites him, and accept this. On the other hand he cannot be a really good lover for you if he does not understand your fantasies, unless of course he happens to *be* your sexual idea.

For example, if your fantasy is one of a gentle, sensuous, romantic lover and he comes on too strong, he will turn you off, no matter how good his lovemaking "technique" is. On the other hand, if his approach is gentle and soft, while you have always secretly yearned to be swept away by a strong, experienced "fatherly" man, lovemaking might be a bit disappointing for both of you, no matter how much you care for each other.

While you are getting to know each other, and becoming intimate, is a great time to talk about your sexual past, your preferences, your desires, and to explore and share your fantasies together. This can be a risk-free first step for two people who are developing an intimate sexual relationship.

Almost everyone has sexual fantasies, but many people feel so guilty that they have never admitted to anyone that they masturbate or that they have erotic fantasies. Therefore it comes as a surprise to many when they find out that these are perfectly normal and commonly experienced by decent and upstanding citizens. Talking about, understanding, and accepting each other's fantasies will deepen the intimacy between you and your partner, and can make your sexual relationship freer and more exciting.

Sexual fantasy can be a great help for monogamous couples seeking to keep their sex lives exciting. I treat a great many couples who have been married for a long time, and who seek help with their sexual problems. It is still startling to me that although they have shared half their lives, have slept in the same bed, have raised children together, have seen each other through many crises, and have known each other intimately in every other area of life, these husbands and wives often do not have the slightest idea of what each other's sexual fantasies are!

An important part of the therapy of such couples is to get them to open up this previously closed and potentially rewarding area of their lives. And in this age of AIDS, open communication with your partner about sex has become extremely important.

A great many people have been brought up to regard sex as dirty or sinful, and many adults still harbor the anti-sexual messages which they received during their early years inside their minds. People raised in very traditional families tend to develop conflicts and feelings of guilt and shame about their sexual feelings and their sexual fantasies. Many men and women feel as if a great weight has been lifted off their shoulders when their old sexual hang-ups are brought out into the open. It is a pleasure to witness the great sense of relief and the deepened feeling of love for their partner which so often occurs when a person finds that he or she is not going to be rejected because of their special sexual desires, even if these are a bit out of the ordinary, or even if they involve persons other than the partner.

You can get a head start on developing this special sexual openness with your partner by exploring your fantasies with him as you are getting to know him, or while you are waiting for the test window to pass or while you are both deciding whether you like each other enough to want to commit yourselves to a sexually exclusive or permanently monogamous relationship.

But revealing and sharing your sexual fantasies is also very nice and intensifies your sexual experience if you just want to "play it safe" in a short-term or nonmonogamous relationship.

Some couples like to tell each other their fantasies while they are stimulating each other or themselves to orgasm in each other's presence, manually or with a vibrator. And for those who have no moral or personal or emotional objections, the sharing of explicit erotic materials, such as Oriental "pillow books,"* and explicit sexual videotapes can be very arousing and gratifying.

Some couples like to stimulate themselves to orgasm while talking about their fantasies to each other by telephone. Each is aroused by the thought that their partner is also getting aroused and coming; they do this for pleasure, not because they are afraid of AIDS. You should be aware that there is nothing quite as safe as telephone sex.

The use of fantasy and erotica is very misunderstood. Many people think that anything other than straight, "missionary position,"† heterosexual fantasies is abnormal. But

---

* Some Oriental cultures regarded sex as an art form and produced books of beautiful erotic drawings, which couples looked at together in bed.
† The face-to-face intercourse position with the man on top and the woman

from a scientific point of view there is nothing inherently sick about any type of sexual fantasy or any sort of erotica. Some people object to pornography because they think it will influence a person to develop perverse sexual desires, or to make him crave violent or sadistic sex. That is not true. Pornographic books, pictures, or films can excite you *only if the scenes tap into already existing fantasies,* which you may not have realized were there, deeply buried in your unconscious. But they were: pornography cannot implant *new* desires into anyone's head. Explicit erotica merely *releases* them and, in fact, pornographic material that does not mesh with your own inner sexual desires will only bore or disgust you.

Actually, fantasies are really "innocent." These mental images have their origin in early childhood, during the development of your sexuality. Sometimes the first things that happened to excite you when you were a small child become "imprinted" and retain their erotic power throughout life. If you peeked at your father taking a shower, or happened to see your parents make love, those kinds of scenes and stories may excite you forever. Sometimes a person's sexual fantasies grow out of his attempts to master his sexual impulses as he grew up within the complicated and often emotionally trying family environment, and these remain permanently in his psyche.

For example, boys whose strict mothers handed out physical punishment may grow up with erotic revenge fantasies of spanking their sexual partner. More often, harshly treated children eroticize these early assaults by their parents and as adults are aroused by the idea of being punished by their partners.

---

beneath and facing him is referred to as the "missionary position" because when Christian missionaries came to some African and Asian countries where the native population was very free about sexual pleasure, the clergymen tried to teach them that anything but the male superior position was wicked and sinful. The Orthodox Judeo-Christian religions even today forbid many of the sexual practices described here, because they are not directly related to reproduction.

I am only talking about what is medically *safe* and *not safe.* You must let your own conscience and sense of morality guide your behavior.

Some people like actually acting out their fantasies, others would hate to actually *do* the things that excite them mentally. As long as you or your partner don't get hurt, it is okay to use, share, and act out your sexual fantasies. Many people have the mistaken belief that having sexual fantasies is a sign of psychological abnormality. That is not the case. Many perfectly normal, decent, and successful people enrich their lives with erotic fantasies. You should also know that just because you and your partner use erotica does not mean that you do not love each other.

Many people think of "real sex" as consisting only of vaginal intercourse. Those who are a bit more worldly might also include oral sex.

But while intercourse is a wonderful experience with the right partner, it is actually not the be-all and end-all of sex for many normal people, and most especially for women. Although they may not always admit this for fear of appearing abnormal, or of hurting their partner's feelings, many women really find foreplay and clitoral stimulation far more enjoyable than penile penetration, and quite a few men secretly prefer masturbation and fantasy and other forms of sexual expression to vaginal intercourse.

Of course, many people do like penetration best. Some women, although not the majority, find nothing as gratifying as the feeling of their lover's hard penis deep inside them, and the favorite fantasy of many men is to come inside the woman they desire.

But even for those people whose first choice is penetration, masturbation and fantasy can be very pleasurable — and it is very much safer than any form of penetration, no matter how protected.

Many men and women do not let themselves enjoy masturbation and fantasy alone or with their partners because they feel guilty about sexual practices that are regarded as sick, kinky, or childish by many in our society. Others secretly enjoy the pleasures of masturbation and fantasy in the privacy of their bedroom, but are too guilty and embarrassed to admit this or suggest sharing these activities with their partners.

But fantasy and parallel self-stimulation or manual stimulation of each other's genitals is the key to safe sex with your partner, and I hope you will not opt for celibacy or condoms, because of some irrational guilt or shame.

However, if you and/or your partner are devout Catholics or Orthodox Jews, fantasy and masturbation are not for you because such activities are forbidden by these religions. These activities might make you feel guilty and conflicted, and could also be destructive to your relationship. You might be much better off remaining celibate until you marry.

We have learned a great deal about the immense erotic potential of shared erotic fantasy and alternative sexual techniques from working with older men who cannot have erections hard enough for penetration because of physical problems. These couples often learn to have wonderful sex by sharing fantasies, oral sex, and improving their skill in stimulating each other manually.

A number of women whose husbands are organically impotent have told me that their marriages and their sexual experiences with their husbands are now more satisfying than ever before.*

You have to be sexually secure to accept erotica as part of your lovemaking. If you are not sure enough of yourself, you will not be able to understand that it is no reflection on your attractiveness or his love for you if your man is turned on by a videotape. You might not be able to accept that he may simply need to focus on fantasy to "tune out" the distraction of trying to please you or worrying about his ability to perform.

By the same token, he shouldn't be threatened if you have an orgasm with your vibrator and not with his penis. He has to be pretty sure of himself as a lover to understand that your using your vibrator does not mean he doesn't turn you on. You would probably need strong clitoral stimulation with any partner.

---

* Men who cannot have firm erections because of such medical problems as diabetes or poor penile circulation may choose to have a penile implant. Many couples are also very satisfied with this procedure.

He may enjoy fantasies that you couldn't enjoy or wouldn't participate in, such as group sex, homosexuality, anal sex, and oral sex, as well as even more unusual things, or he may get excited by the fantasy of sex with another woman.

Do not be jealous. He is in bed with *you*, not with her.

By accepting his fantasy, you can let him know that you are not putting him down, and that you genuinely want him to have pleasure, but you are not going to take part in things that arouse him if they are not to your taste.

I do not mean to imply that the use of sexual fantasy is always healthy or constructive. Some people use fantasy like alcohol; they escape into their erotic imagery as a way of detaching themselves from their partner. But this is not as often the case as people think.

The reason that I have dwelled in such detail on sexual fantasy is that fantasy, together with manual genital stimulation and sensuous touching, is the key to *great safe sex*. This is especially important for women who do not want to limit themselves to sex with one man, or for those who are simply not ready for a lifetime commitment, but who do not wish to give up sex and romance. I do not want you to miss out on these risk-free forms of sexual gratification with your partner simply because you have mistaken ideas about what is "normal" and what is "sick."

CONDOMS AGAIN

Condoms are an excellent means of reducing the risks under certain circumstances, but only if you make that choice with the full realization that infected fluids can seep out over the rim of the condom, or remain on his moist pubic hair and yours, or seep out of his penis before he puts on his condom or after he removes it. Also keep in mind that semen is *not* the only body fluid that contains AIDS virus particles and infected cells. These are also likely to be present in his saliva, pre-ejaculatory secretions and on his mucous membranes, and you can get AIDS even if the condom does not break or does not have any visible holes in it.

You must understand that you are taking an unknown but significant degree of risk and that this risk is greater than the dry sexual activities I have described above. But if intercourse is your main desire, and you are very attracted to him, you might choose to take the risk.

Or, if you are in a monogamous relationship with a man who might have been exposed, and his first test has come out okay, you might want to use condoms with spermicides until he is retested six months later, as recommended by Dr. Theresa Crenshaw, the chairperson of the task force on AIDS of the American Association of Sex Educators, Counselors, and Therapists.

IF ONE PARTNER IS INFECTED AND THE OTHER IS NOT

If your partner is infected and you want to completely eliminate the risks of becoming infected, celibacy is foolproof! But the extremely low-risk dry sex activities that were described in this chapter are also very reasonable choices.

With a partner known to be an AIDS virus carrier, I would consider the 20 or 30 percent risk of using condoms too high, especially for women of child-bearing age. However, there are times in life when one takes risks and other times when one doesn't. All doctors can do, or should do, is to give you the true facts, so that you and your partners can make informed choices.

If both of you are seropositive, you probably have nothing to lose. Do what you like to do with each other, but *please do not have sex with an uninfected person, even with condoms!* That is tantamount to murder.*

---

* Some people feel it is okay for a person with HIV infection to have sex with a healthy partner as long as he or she informs the person. I disagree. If you

SAFE DRY SEX IS NOT SO TERRIBLE FOR WOMEN

The restraints required to make sex safe are actually a pretty good deal from the standpoint of female sexuality. As it turns out, the sexual activities that will eliminate the risk of infection for you as well as for him are not as objectionable to most women as they are to many men. In fact, some of the "safe" erotic activities are actually preferred to "unsafe" sexual intercourse by many women.

Dry safe sex (except for not being able to kiss your lover without fear) comes pretty close to what my generation used to call "making out," and what the textbooks term "foreplay."

Many married women experienced much more pleasure from being touched, kissed, and fondled, often to orgasm, which was the custom for engaged couples before the "sexual revolution," than they felt from vaginal intercourse later. In those days most brides were virgins, and for many, the first experience with actual intercourse on the honeymoon was disappointing. They had had a great deal of pleasure from "making out," but "going all the way" was not all that wonderful.

Women often complain that they do not have enough time to get aroused because their partners rush through these (dry and safe) preliminaries in their eagerness to proceed with (wet and risky) genital penetration.

But remember, manual stimulation of the clitoris, which is also in the low-risk category, is the *only* way 75 percent of normal women can reach orgasm. In sexual therapy I have seen many an insecure husband who is upset by his inability to give her an orgasm with his penis pressure his wife and spoil her pleasure as well as his own by desperately trying to "hold out" until she comes. These men need to

---

inform someone you are going to kill him, and he agrees, you are still guilty of murder.

learn that clitoral eroticism is a normal female response pattern, that it certainly does not mean that a wife does not love her husband, and that, although many women pretend otherwise, only about 25 percent of women are able to climax on penetration alone, and over 70% of perfectly normal women require "clitoral assistance."*

Foreplay and clitoral stimulation are dry safe sex activities which women enjoy and which are very much "in" today. Although by far the great majority of men are eager ·to be good lovers and enjoy seeing their women have pleasure, some have acted as though foreplay and clitoral stimulation were doing the woman a favor. He may have made you feel that this was some unpleasant homework he had to do before he got his "dessert." Now that it is for his own safety as well as yours, perhaps your lover might be more enthusiastic.

An extra little benefit of the "safe sex" era for those women who are aroused intensely by using vibrators or who need vibrator stimulation to have an orgasm is that it has become more acceptable to use a vibrator.

Secure men have always accepted and encouraged this, and enjoyed sharing their partner's pleasure. Others are threatened and feel competitive with those little machines, and they make their women feel too embarrassed to use this form of stimulation in their presence. But genital stimulation with a vibrator is safe and dry and it is now okay to use one.

Be sure to use your own and keep it clean and disinfected. Do not let him use his vibrator unless you are absolutely sure he has not used it with anyone else. You can give yourself an orgasm in your partner's presence and/or he might also enjoy your using his vibrator to stimulate his genitalia.

Last but not least for women, the age of AIDS has brought with it a greater emphasis on monogamy and exclusive sexual relationships. Men are now more willing to

* Scientific References, Group VIII: Sex Therapy and Sexology.

commit themselves to a relationship and to making it work, rather than risk playing sexual Russian roulette in various bedrooms, or choosing the unpleasant alternative of a lonely sexless life.

Sexually exclusive relationships and earlier marriages are on the rise, and fidelity is getting a break, because married people will have to think twice before they try to "fix" their unsatisfactory sex lives the "quick and easy way," with extramarital sex. Men and women who want good sex will now have to make deeper commitments to improving their relationships, rather than risk catching the AIDS virus from a prostitute or a stranger.

I am already seeing these trends in my office as increasing numbers of couples with marital problems and/or "boring" or ungratifying sex lives are seeking help together to resolve their differences. The process, of course, can only work if both spouses are equally committed to improving the sexual aspect of their relationships.

The new interest in monogamy is hardly likely to raise loud protests from most women.

That is not to say that these changes in our sexual behavior in the age of AIDS are all to the disadvantage of men. Men will also benefit from the freedom from performance pressures and from the more open communication about sex which are emerging because of men's and women's caution about AIDS.

6

How to Say No to Sex
Until It Is Safe
Without Losing Your Man

The great majority of American women should have no problem avoiding exposure to AIDS without having to give up sex and romance if they follow these simple rules:

1. Do not have sex or only engage in safe dry sex (see Chapter 5) until you *know* that your partner is not infected.
2. You can make love in any way that you and your lover prefer, with no risk at all, safely, wet or dry, condom or no condom, if you make certain that he is not infected with the AIDS virus, and if you are sure he is not being exposed to AIDS by sleeping with anyone else.

Of course if you remain celibate you avoid the risks of sexually transmitted AIDS entirely.

But women in this country do not have to forgo sex, love, or romance to keep safe, as long as they are smart about it.

You can confine your sex life to one man whose negative AIDS status you are sure of, or you can feel free to have sex with more than one partner if you limit yourself to the safe, dry sexual activites described in the previous chapter.

Which path you choose is a personal and moral decision, not a medical one.

The circumstances of women in this age of AIDS vary widely. However, whether you are single or married, old or young, rich or poor, white, brown, black, or yellow, if you follow these basic rules and use your intuition and your good common sense, it should be easy for most of you to keep safe without losing your partners or giving up love and romance in the process.

COMMUNICATING WITH YOUR PARTNER

To find out if your partner is in the high-risk category — if he is bisexual, or shoots drugs, or sleeps with prostitutes— you have to ask some pretty personal questions. How can you possibly do that, and also hold off on sex, without turning off every date? And won't insisting that he get tested ruin your relationship? And how can you raise such personal and embarrassing issues as masturbation and fantasy, which you must do if you want to stick to safe sex, without making him think you are weird?

You have to be gracious and tactful and straightforward. If on your first date you quiz him like a schoolteacher about his sexual activities in the last ten years, or if you immediately ask him if he has ever used intravenous drugs, or if you take out your note pad to write down the date of the blood transfusion he had after his car accident, or if you inquire about the details of what kind of women he has slept with and how many there have been in the last ten years, you will not get the truth. But you will not get the AIDS virus from him either, because he is not likely to stick around.

But remember, men also are worried about AIDS today. Maybe he is more scared than you are. He may not mind your honesty and openness and courage in bringing up such personal, sexual matters. In fact, he may actually be relieved that you saved him the trouble of speaking up, and appreciative that you care about your safety and his. He might respect you and feel closer to you, but only if you do this nicely and with sensitivity.

Dr. Michael Marmor of the New York University Medical Center makes the excellent point that while ". . . women should take special precautions to avoid bisexual men and I.V. drug users, they need to know how to ask about *risk-laden exposures*, and not just about how people label themselves." He suggests that a woman not ask a potential lover if he is bisexual. "You should inquire if he has ever had sex with another man, even just once, at any time since 1977. The same holds true for I.V. drug use. Don't ask, 'Are you an addict?' but, 'Have you tried intravenous drugs even once since 1977?' A positive answer means that he needs to be tested before you can assume he is free of HIV infection."

But remember, no matter how great your communication skills are, some people lie. So information alone is not enough. You also have to get to know your partner well enough and use your instincts and learn to "read" *the feelings he evokes in you* to judge what kind of person he is. Can you trust him? Is he the type who would knowingly risk your life and your future for the sake of one night's pleasure? I would venture that intuition, intimacy, and good common sense have a lower failure rate than condoms alone.

Here are some guidelines on getting a true drug and sex history to determine whether your partner could have been exposed, and/or should be tested before you have sex with him.

MEN TO WORRY ABOUT

1. *Bisexual Men*

For the great majority of American women the highest risk by far of getting infected with the AIDS virus is from having sex with bisexual men who have been infected by homosexual exposure.

Unless they live in a drug-infested inner-city ghetto, where sex with an addict is the greatest danger, most white and middle-class women are not going to socialize and sleep with I.V. drug users. But bisexuality is much more common among men than people realize, and women who live in neighborhoods in and surrounding the high-risk areas where the AIDS virus is prevalent might very well unknowingly become exposed to AIDS through bisexual men who have had homosexual experiences. Catching the AIDS virus from a bisexual man is also a danger for women who make love to strangers they meet on vacations in areas frequented by gay and bisexual men—for example, Fire Island, Zurich, Key West, and Haiti.

Exclusively gay men are no danger to you because they are not interested in having sex with you, but we have known since Kinsey's survey in 1948 that there are many more bisexual men than men who are exclusively homosexual.* And please be aware that many men who have bisexual proclivities have strong desires for women as well as for men.

It is impossible for you to know whether or not the new man in your life has had homosexual experiences in the last eight or ten years. Some gay or bisexual men are obviously effeminate, but others are virile, masculine, and athletic and there is no way to tell a man's sexual proclivities from his behavior or appearance. Not even professionals can be certain if a man has had homosexual exposure. And at this time when homosexuality has become so dangerous, we are seeing growing numbers of bisexual and homosexual men who are seeking therapy to overcome their sexual aversions to women, and to increase their capacity for heterosexual gratification.

I have a good deal of clinical experience with helping men who are dissatisfied with their homosexual orientation to overcome their aversion to heterosexual sex. Many of

* Scientific References, Group VIII: Sex Therapy and Sexology.

these men have been trying to find out if they can enjoy sex with a woman on their own, and often without being tested for AIDS first. It is only natural that they tend to pick gentle, supportive, sensitive women who are not likely to hurt them.

A man with a bisexual or a homosexual history is going to be self-protective just like anyone else. He is not likely to admit his homosexual experiences to you. He wants to avoid being rejected or humiliated by you, and if he has been "in the closet," you cannot blame him for not wanting to risk exposure. However, if he is a decent person he will have been avoiding homosexual encounters for at least one year, and have had himself tested and cleared before he makes love to you, but you cannot count on that.

2. I.V. Drug Users

I.V. drug users are very dangerous for poor and disadvantaged women who live in one of the large drug-infested urban communities, such as those in the New York City metropolitan area or Miami, where drug abuse is extremely common. It has been estimated that 80 percent of I.V. drug using males have wives or girlfriends who do not use drugs. Black and Hispanic women and female street prostitutes are particularly likely to be victimized, and not enough is being done to protect these vulnerable groups.

According to research carried out by epidemiologists Ann Hardy and Mary Guinan on 2000 reported cases of AIDS in females, 70 percent of AIDS cases in women occurred among blacks and Hispanics. Unhappily, a woman who is black is 13 times as likely as one who is white to fall victim, and 90 percent of infants born with AIDS are black. We certainly have not done enough to protect minority women and children.

I.V. drug users sometimes have needle scars on the inner surface of their forearms but some do not, so you can't rely on this sign and it is often difficult to figure out if a man is a user.

If he is from your own community, you might know who

deals and who goes to "shooting galleries," and you will be doing yourself a great big favor if you keep these gentlemen out of your bed.

Even if he swears to you that he has kicked the habit, you know how difficult that is, and unless he is enrolled in a legitimate drug rehabilitation program, say no to him!

But if you have a relationship with an I.V. drug abuser and you love him and do not want to stop seeing him, at least ask him to get tested. If he is not yet infected make sure that he never uses anyone else's needle, even if it means you have to buy hypodermics for him!

I.V. drug abusers who do not share needles pose *no* special risks to their sexual partners. It is not the *drug* that will make you ill but your partner's sharing his needles, because he is likely to have been infected by injecting himself with hypodermic needles which are full of AIDS-laden blood.

The likelihood that an addict is seropositive varies greatly by geographic area. In some places the odds that he is infected could be as high as 70 to 80 percent. If it turns out that your man is a drug user and infected, and you want to continue to have sexual intercourse with him, you have no alternative to using condoms to reduce the risk.

3. Men Who Have Become Infected with AIDS by Sleeping with High-Risk Women

Probably less than 1 percent of "Johns"* are HIV carriers at this time. But this pool of infection is rising rapidly, and these men present a great danger for the "average" unfaithful American housewife and the normal sexually active single woman who live in rural and small-town America, where the prevalence of infection is otherwise extremely low.

Avoid having sex with men who frequent prostitutes. Prostitutes risk infection both from their customers and also from their own not uncommon addiction to I.V.

---

* A "John" is a prostitute's customer.

drugs. Prostitutes are often caught in a vicious circle which puts them at high risk for becoming drug addicts, and hence victims of AIDS. These women often begin to use drugs to dull their feelings of disgust when they have to have sex with unappealing customers. Then they get hooked. After that they need the income from selling sex to support their habit. Others become addicted first, and then turn to prostitution to pay for the drugs.

The risk of a man's contracting AIDS from a prostitute varies widely and depends on the prevalence of AIDS in the town where she works. For example, one study found that 18.7 percent of those female prostitutes tested in Miami, Florida, and 57.1 percent* in the Newark/Jersey City/Paterson area of New Jersey were infected in 1987, while none of the prostitutes who were sampled from a "low risk" area like Las Vegas were infected (see Table 2 in Chapter 1).

Therefore, men who travel to high-risk areas and who might have sex with high-risk women there, are far more dangerous than men who stay put in low-risk communities. Sailors who go on shore at African ports and men who frequently visit high-risk areas are potentially dangerous for you.

In general, promiscuous men are more dangerous than men who are monogamous because the risks of infection get progressively higher when a person has sexual exposures with more partners.

There are some people, more often men than women, who have a compulsive drive to have sex. They have been called "sexual addicts," and they are more likely to have been exposed and are therefore more dangerous. I am not sure whether people really become addicted to sex, in the same sense as they become addicted to alcohol or heroin. At the last meeting of the American Psychiatric Association Committee on Psychosexual Dysfunctions, of which I am

* Frighteningly, a study done in 1985 showed a figure for Newark of 24 percent. A high figure even then, and see how dramatically it has risen in just two years.

a member, a group of experts on human sexuality con-
cluded that there is not sufficient evidence to say that there
actually is such a disorder as sexual "addiction" in the true
sense of the word. We thought that perhaps many people
who are guilty about their natural sexual feelings label
themselves "sick" or "addicted."

But there certainly are individuals, again more often
men than women, who are totally preoccupied with sex,
and who become extremely uncomfortable if they do not
have frequent sexual outlets. These sexually compulsive
individuals often crave sex with multiple partners. Sexually
compulsive men will give you grief even if they do not give
you AIDS, but now you have an extra reason to avoid
them.

4. Artificial Insemination

The semen of HIV carriers is infectious and several women
have contracted AIDS from a *single artificial insemination
exposure* from an infected donor. Therefore be *sure* you
ask your fertility doctor to screen the *donor* for AIDS antibodies before you proceed with insemination.

FOR GAY WOMEN

Sexually active women who are exclusively lesbian have sex
with other women who also tend to avoid sex with men.
Therefore the risk of acquiring AIDS through sexual transmission is extremely low.

However, one case of probable female-to-female sexual
transmission has been reported.

In an article published in the *Annals of Internal Medicine* in 1986, Dr. Michael Marmor described a twenty-
five-year-old lesbian I.V. drug abuser who infected her
twenty-six-year-old female lover with AIDS, possibly by
way of an exchange of menstrual blood during sex. Thus,
even though sexual transmission is extremely unlikely be-

tween women, lesbians also should know their partners' AIDS status, especially if they are drug users or call girls.

THE NEW RULES OF BEDROOM ETIQUETTE

Give yourself the time to establish a relationship and get to really know your man.

Then the first thing you should do is to find out if he knows the true facts about safe and unsafe sex. Bring up the topic gently. Make sure your timing is right. If he does not know what is safe and what is not, if he thinks condoms are safe, if he does not understand that you can get infected from oral sex, educate him, show him the way.

Maybe I am naive, but I honestly believe that most men will not act immorally once they have their consciences raised about the danger into which they may be placing you, especially after they learn to care more about you as a person than just a sexual opportunity. But I wouldn't gamble my life on that.

Males are only human, and if a man is strongly attracted to you, if he wants to make love to you very badly, or even if he just wants to "score," you can't count on him to be honest about his sexual history. He may not tell you that he has been promiscuous and/or had sex with high-risk women. You also can't count on his admitting, when you meet him at a singles bar or at an office party or at your cousin's wedding, that he uses I.V. drugs. If he wants to go to bed with you badly enough, he is not likely to tell you anything that will dissuade you.

Moreover, everyone has the tendency to deny that they are in danger. We all want to sweep unpleasant and threatening things under the rug. If he has been exposed he may want to put it out of his mind, *he himself might not want to know if he is infected.* So if he has a silent HIV infection, the chances are he does not even know it, and if he has been taken in by the condom propaganda, he may honestly not realize he is putting you in any danger.

It is up to you to protect yourself. But be warm and

sensitive to his feelings. You have a much better chance of learning the truth if you make him feel secure. Make it clear that you will not reject him if he has been exposed (if it is true that you will not), that the only reason you want him to be tested and cleared before you have sex is so that you won't get ill. And tell him that you too are willing to be tested for his protection.

How can you do this without offending him and embarrassing yourself?

Every man and every woman is a unique individual with his or her own special sexual desires, anxieties, vulnerabilities, hopes and dreams for love and romance, and moral values. Therefore it is really not possible to give you a single script or a formula that will guide you in approaching your prospective partner in the right way. You will have to write your own script, but perhaps some typical scenarios will help you.

For example, you are twenty-seven years old, and you have just broken up with your boyfriend. You are lonely and looking for a new romance. You are sharing a summer house at the shore with a bunch of friends, and your roommate brings her handsome, curly-haired, sensitive, brilliant cousin who has just graduated from Harvard Law School out for the weekend. He is attracted to you, you are attracted to him. It is a beautiful starry night. Everyone else who is sharing the house is married or engaged and paired up.

Now what?

Three years ago, you might have gone to bed with him. Now you really can't.

You have to honestly tell him that you too are attracted to him and would really want to make love to him but you have just met each other and you are afraid of AIDS.

If he tells you that he's going to use a condom, you know that he doesn't know the facts, and you will have to educate him before you go any further. You will also have to let him know that you would like to get to know him much better before you make love to him and you hope he feels the same way too.

If he is decent and not self-destructive and not sexually driven, and if he is really interested in you, he will not take offense. But he will be turned off if you come on too strong and aggressive. If you give him the message that you suspect that he's untrustworthy, or question his masculinity, or if you come across as an obsessive, controlling hypo-chondriac, I would not blame him for losing interest.

But if you are direct and gentle and warm, and he is a nice, sensible person, an open, honest discussion of the dangers of AIDS that you both face might actually get your relationship started off on an intimate, honest level. And that is a very good start.

Suppose that three weeks later he admits to you that he experimented with homosexuality five years ago in college. Please do not reject him on that account alone. A man's having had or having homosexual feelings does not neces-sarily mean he is neurotic or incapable of loving a woman. True, he could be basically ambivalent about women and big trouble for you. But he also could turn out to be sensi-tive and caring and a wonderful partner for you. Appreci-ate his courage. His honesty is a gift to you. But for heaven's sake, do not let him talk you into having unsafe sex with him until he has been tested and cleared.

If a man gives you a hard time when you say no to instant sex, if he makes you feel guilty, if he asks "Don't you trust me?" or "Are you suggesting that I am a junkie?" or if he says "So you think I'm gay," or if he threatens to leave, or calls you neurotic — *do not back down*. Sticking to your position when a man will not take no for an answer is the most difficult part for a "nice" woman. It is extremely hard for a gentle woman to step out of her "good girl" role and stand up to a man she likes, and who really wants sex with her. It will be even more difficult if he plays on your guilt. No feeling woman wants to hurt or frustrate a man. But you have to learn to be self-protective. Your life depends on it.

Here is another typical scenario:

You are forty-three, recently divorced, insecure about entering the dating world again after twenty years. You have had no sex with anyone for the past year and a half, but the wounds have healed enough for you to start socializing. All the men you have met so far have been nerds.

Miraculously you meet an eligible man at a friend's dinner party. You are told he is successful. He is attractive, intelligent, worldly, and he takes you home in his convertible. He invites himself up to your apartment for a drink, you let him, and he makes a pass.

You tell him to slow down.

How can you do that nicely? (Because you certainly want to see him again.)

He is aggressive and won't take no for an answer. (But you don't want a passive man, do you?)

He asks you in a hurt voice, "You don't think I'm one of those gay guys, do you?" And proceeds to tell you about his sexual prowess. Although you are a bit offended, you reassure him that you find him very masculine and that was the furthest thought from your mind. He then implies that you are too nervous for him and you are not the only fish in the sea. He also unbalances you by asking pointedly how old your children are.

Maybe he is an aggressive "chauvinist pig" who just wants to "get laid." If so, good riddance.

But maybe he is not. Maybe he is as sensitive to rejection as you are. Maybe he too has been hurt and maybe he is trying in his own way, without appearing to be weak, to see if your AIDS story is just a subtle way of rejecting him.

If that's what is really going on, if he is really a vulnerable man who has been hurt and has developed a tough outer crust, then reassure him that you are not trying to manipulate or tease him. That you feel badly about saying no. That you really like him and find him attractive. Also you should let him know that you are not a prude and that you like sex (if this is true). If you really want to catch his interest you could be open and tell him about some past pleasurable sexual experiences you have had, and even suggest that you could be interested in some safe sex with him one of these days, when you get to know each other a little better. But you have to be firm that you are not going to bed with anyone, even with Paul Newman or Bruce Springsteen, unless you get to know them very well first.

It will also heighten your conflict if he manipulates you with flattery. No woman wants to risk losing the admiration of a man who makes her feel desired and beautiful.

It is especially hard to say no to a man whom you truly love. But think, if he returns your love he will want to protect you and make you comfortable, and he will understand that your reason for wanting to stick to safe sex has nothing to do with any cruelty on your part, or any lack of desire.

You are not likely to ruin your relationship by waiting for sex until you feel safe, if you are open and reassure him that you are not rejecting him, and that you care for him and trust him (if this is true) but you want to get to know him better, and that you would like an exclusive sexual relationship with him for your protection and his.

If he admits that he may have been exposed, because he has had homosexual experiences, slept with prostitutes, or used hard drugs in the past, tell him that you do not think less of him (if it is true that you do not). You simply feel vulnerable, there is so much at stake for you, and you need the reassurance that he can easily give you by taking the test even if he thinks it is not necessary. If he is worried about possible repercussions, he can take the test at an alternate testing site.

A decent man will respect a woman's right to protect herself and he will think more of you if you pursue this matter in a gentle and sensitive way, especially if he cares for you.* But if he still refuses, if he pushes you to have sex despite your fears, if he will not discuss safe sex with you in an open way, or if he puts you down when you bring up this subject, which is after all for *the benefit of both of you*, let him go.

* See Appendix F.

How to Bring up Safe Sex

It might be very embarrassing for many women to bring up the specifics of "safe sex." This is especially difficult for women in their forties, fifties, sixties, and older (yes, older women do have sex), who grew up before the new sexual freedom.

If you are interested in getting closer to him I suggest that you first bring up the topic of safe sex intellectually, and not wait until you are already in the bedroom, where this is much more threatening.

For example:

He is driving you home from a lovely dinner. You can see that he wants to make love to you. You also want physical closeness, but of course you want to stay healthy. You might ask, "What is your idea of safe sex?" and then listen to him.

If he is too afraid of AIDS to do *anything* physical, and you would like him to, you can open his eyes to the fact that there are lots of nice dry safe sex things you could enjoy together.

If he thinks condoms are safe, straighten him out.

If you are both too uncomfortable to talk about masturbation and fantasy, admit to him that you are extremely embarrassed, and that you do not want him to think badly of you, and tell him you have a *book that explains what is medically safe and what is risky*, and let him read Chapter 4 which explains how the virus is transmitted through various forms of sex, and also Chapter 5, on safe dry sex. That way he can blame anything that offends him on me and on this book, and not you. But if it is helpful, and it breaks the ice, you get the credit.

Actually, the fear of AIDS gives you something important in common which really forces you to communicate on a genuine and intimate level. Your relationship will be off to a good start if you handle this with dignity and sensitivity.

For Married Women

If you have been married or living with a man for ten or more years, providing he is not a drug abuser, has not received infected blood, is not in the health field and exposed to AIDS patients, is not bisexual, and you know him well enough to trust that he has not had sex outside of your relationship, the risks are so *negligible* that you do not have anything to worry about and you should just go about your life and enjoy sex together.

But if you have any reason to suspect that your husband or your steady partner might have been exposed, the same rules for eliminating the risks that should guide the behavior of sexually active single women apply to you.

Approximately 60 percent of married American men and 40 percent of married American women have had at least one extramarital relationship, and the spouse usually never finds out. So you might not be completely paranoid if you suspect that he has strayed, even though he has the reputation of being the most faithful husband in town. But the chances are also very good that you are completely wrong about your suspicions, and you should be prepared for both possibilities. And remember, even if he has been playing around a little, especially if his girlfriends have been "low risk," the chances that he has been infected are still very remote, probably less than one in thirty thousand.

However, if you think there is really something to worry about, if you sense that perhaps he is secretly bisexual, or sleeping with high-risk women, *you have to speak up.*

For example, you are in your early forties. You have been married for twenty years and have three children and you have always thought that you and your husband have a better than average marriage. But last week your best friend wept her heart out to you because she had just found out that her husband has been having an affair with his secretary. She was blaming herself for hiding her head in the sand, because she now realized that her husband had avoided sex with her for the past year and a half.

You suddenly become aware of the fact that you and your husband, who travels a great deal on business, have had less and less sex in the past few years and that it is now down to only once a month. You suddenly wake up to the fact that you are vulnerable. But you are afraid to face him. If he has been faithful, he will feel hurt and angry at your lack of trust in him, and if you raise the question of *his* infidelity, he might also become suspicious that you have been having an affair.

Need I say if *you* have been "playing around," unless you are absolutely certain that your lover is safe, it is *your moral obligation to your husband to have yourself tested.*

The risks of catching AIDS from an affair were really tiny ten years ago. They are still small, but each passing year the prevalence of the virus is increasing, and so is the risk of heterosexual transmission.

To put it more simply, if you had an affair with a stranger in this country six years ago, the chances of your becoming infected might have been less than one in one million (0.0001 percent). Last year they could have been one in thirty thousand (0.01 percent), *one hundred times* more likely, but still very small.

If you are at all afraid that word of your test might get around, you do not have to take it in your hometown, and you do not have to give your name if you have access to an alternate testing site. But it is terribly unfair to your husband if you do not protect him from exposure.

When you confront your husband, if he really has been having sex on the outside he is apt to feel so guilty that he might get even angrier and more defensive. But you have to speak up. If you hold your doubts inside, your anger will build up and eventually it will come out in a way that might be destructive to your marriage. Put your fears aside. Maybe he will get angry, but he has been angry before and he will forgive you. Besides, maybe it is time to start talking about improving your sex life together.

Tell him you believe and trust him (if this is true). Tell him that you are probably completely wrong but your

HOW TO SAY NO TO SEX WITHOUT LOSING YOUR MAN

friend's dilemma has upset you (if this is true). But you feel very vulnerable and concerned and you need him to protect and understand you and get tested even if he thinks it is not necessary. Be gentle. Be sensitive to his feelings. Put the priority on your *relationship*, not on your *ego* or your *wounded pride*.

Do not push him "underground" by threatening him. Even if you are right and have every reason to be angry, you will not learn the truth unless you are very sensitive about how difficult it might be for him to admit that he had been cheating or that he had been hiding his homosexuality or his drug habit from you. And he will never tell you, unless you can reassure him that if he tells the truth you will not reject him.

Before you ask him point-blank if he has cheated, prepare the ground by raising his consciousness to the dangers of AIDS virus exposure. He would probably feel terrible if he unknowingly gave you AIDS, and he might simply have pushed that possibility out of his mind.

Let's look at another hypothetical scenario:

You live in a medium-sized town in Pennsylvania. You have been married for ten years to a wonderful man whom you love. You do not have sex all that frequently, but when you do it is fine. You are organizing his closet while he is on one of his monthly overnight business trips to New York City, and you come across a large collection of male homosexual magazines, which had been hidden under some sweaters on the top shelf. The magazines are filled with explicit pictures of attractive men making love to each other or masturbating. You are shocked and outraged, and you then panic about AIDS.

Do you have anything to worry about? You bet you have.

Statistically, the only real danger that a long-time steady partner will infect you is if he has secret homosexual encounters. If you are lucky, he expresses the homosexual side of his sexuality only in fantasy. That is common, and perfectly safe for both of you. But it is also very common for bisexual married men to have homosexual encounters outside of their marriage, and they usually do this outside their own communities.

If he is in *love* with a man, you have a serious marital problem, apart from possibly having been exposed to the AIDS virus. But if he has just had impersonal homosexual encounters, and your relationship is basically sound, and if you can find it in your heart to accept his bisexual feelings, it is entirely possible that you and he can continue to have a very good marriage and sex life. Do not overreact. Such marriages often get better and more intimate once his secret interest in men becomes an open issue. But only if you can *accept* this, not just *tolerate* it. You may need professional help as a couple to accomplish this. I have seen many mutually gratifying marriages between heterosexual women and bisexual men, and it usually helps if the husband can express his homosexual desires through fantasy shared with his wife. I have also seen some bisexual men who are wonderful fathers to boys and to girls. And I have also seen some disasters. Do not prejudge. Use your head and your heart.

In any case, make absolutely sure you and he are tested and cleared, and that he has truly given up his homosexual contact with men, before you have sex with him again.

In terms of the relationship, it is extremely important for women who are worried about being exposed through their partners to volunteer to also have themselves tested even though, unless you have been playing around with high-risk males, the chances that either of you are infected are almost nil. But fair is fair. He is also entitled to protection and it will make it easier for him to take the test if you also volunteer and you do it together as a couple.

THE NEW SEXUAL MORALITY

It is up to you and your partner to *do unto others as you would have others do unto you*. Translated into sex that means that if you have been exposed it is your moral obligation to have yourself tested to find out if your exposure has resulted in infection. If you have had (wet) sex with anyone, and if you turn out to be infected, and again, even though this is highly unlikely for most of you, it is incumbent upon you to inform your partner, so he too can have himself tested to find out what his AIDS status is. Truth and decency and honest communication together with testing are the cornerstone of the prevention of the sexual chain reaction that could easily result in a widespread AIDS epidemic.

You have to feel good enough about yourself to feel entitled to protect yourself. But you also have to know how to say no to unsafe sex until you *know* he is not infected — without losing a valued relationship, without hurting his feelings, without being defensive, without sitting home alone, and without ruining your marriage.

You will only be able to assert yourself effectively if your self-esteem is high enough for you to feel *entitled* not to let yourself be used or hurt.

Many women need professional help to become appropriately assertive and self-protective. But look out! Some therapists, sex counselors, and sex therapists are misinformed and biased about AIDS, and may give you poor advice. If you go for help and hear the therapist say, "Forget it, you are too insecure, you are merely trying to avoid intimacy, just use a condom," ask the therapist, "Just exactly what level of protection do condoms provide for women?" See what he or she answers before you take any advice.

Dr. Theresa Crenshaw has organized some excellent women's self-help, assertiveness, and AIDS educational groups on the West Coast. If you need help or want information about organizing such a group, write to her.*

* Theresa L. Crenshaw, M.D., The Crenshaw Clinic, 550 Washington, San Diego, CA 92103.

7

Lysistrata:
Women's Strike
Against AIDS

Lysistrata, a play by Aristophanes first performed in ancient Greece in 411 B.C., shows the power of women to act together to protect their families and their communities.

The drama enacts the story of an Athenian woman, Lysistrata, who more than 2400 years ago became frustrated by the needless deaths and mutilations of sons and husbands, by the years of lonely waiting while the men were off to battle, by food shortages, corruptions, and all the assorted outrages and miseries that were produced by the unending wars between the city-states of ancient Greece. She called together the women of Athens and those of Sparta, Athens' adversary, and also women from the other regions that had joined the war, and organized the first documented and successful women's strike for peace.

Lysistrata's plan was simple and effective. The women agreed that they would all withhold sex from their combative husbands until they stopped the fighting. The men, first furious, then cajoling, later flattering and guilt-provoking, got nowhere. So they ultimately gave in and declared a truce. Thus peace finally settled over the land. Then everyone had a big party, and went home happily to make love.

Aristophanes' ancient erotic and comical political satire is a fitting parable for our time of AIDS.

We women form the "bridge" that is virtually the only avenue by which the AIDS virus can escape from its current confinement to the small, highly concentrated pool of infected high-risk men and spread out to the general population, which is still largely uncontaminated.

By virtue of our strategic position in this sexually transmitted disease women have the power and the obligation to guard the general population from the coming infestation. Our bodies form a protective ring around the breeding grounds of the AIDS virus. The barrier of women is fragile and no one is helping to fortify us. But if we don't do it no one will.

The AIDS virus can get out of the infected reservoir into mainsteam America only through our bodies. We can close the bridge if, like Lysistrata's union of women, we do not have sex with infected males. We must form an impenetrable barrier. We must not let the virus use our sexual organs, which were meant to bring forth life, to kill our children, our families, and ultimately everyone. We must use our heads, not our emotions, to keep the epidemic within its present bounds until it burns itself out, or until the scientists find a remedy.

Young girls in our high schools and junior high schools who are just becoming sexually active are the most vulnerable and the most penetrable part of the bridge, and prevention efforts and consciousness-raising should concentrate on these youngsters. We must as a society teach our daughters the importance of avoiding exposure, of eliminating the risks of infection, as far as this is possible. This is our duty to ourselves and to society.

We have to give our daughters the message that they must say no to casual sex. "Sorry kids, it was fun for a while, but those carefree days of meeting a guy at a party and going home with him to bed are gone. Now you have to confine your sexual experiences to monogamous relationships or insist on safe dry sex only. But that is not really all that terrible. It won't hurt you to wait until you get to know a boy and trust him not to hurt you before you make love."

Every child should continue to receive the "message" that sex is wonderful and natural in order to develop into a sexually healthy adult, free of hang-ups. But we must also warn our youngsters that it is dangerous to have sex with an infected man. They must understand that if they become infected they will then infect heterosexual, drug-free men who are still at low risk. This will start a chain reaction that will end in a tragic epidemic.

T.S. Eliot was prophetic when he wrote, "This is the way the world ends, not with a bang, but a whimper."* In this age of AIDS there is a real danger that the world as we know it might end not with a nuclear bang, but with the whimpers of dying AIDS patients.

Our current public health policy, which relies mainly on risk reduction with condoms, is not good enough for adolescents. We want to close those bridges *completely*, not just partially. *Risk avoidance* and *elimination* should be our primary goal for women, with risk reduction and condoms definitely a second-line defense.

For heaven's sake, parents, teachers, sex educators, and politicians: *Stop giving out condoms to the kids! Stop falsely reassuring them that it's okay to have sex as long as you use a condom!* That is a lie with lethal consequences for all of us.

We also must increase our efforts to teach our kids the extreme danger of using drugs and especially of sharing needles.

Unfortunately, 27 percent of men who are carriers are heterosexually active I.V. drug users and bisexuals, and

---

* *The Hollow Men,* by T.S. Eliot.

therein lies our greatest danger. We must give our girls the message *never, never, never, never* to have anything but the *safest sex,* or better yet, *no sex at all,* unless she knows her partner well and they have an *exclusive relationship.*

Every young woman must know for certain that her partner has not been exposed, and if he has, she must make sure that he is *tested and cleared* before she has sex with him and then only if she can trust that he is not having sex with anyone else. Many people, especially the men, will object to a return to monogamy and exclusive sexual relationships, and some may complain about the limitations of *dry* sex. I can understand that, but the alternatives are unacceptable to women until we have a cure. Sexually active women who wish to prevent pregnancy should go back to barrier contraception (condoms and diaphragms) because of the additional advantage of reducing the risk of exposure to AIDS. But we will only be successful in closing the bridge of heterosexual transmission completely if our educational programs start emphasizing the need to *eliminate* the risks of sexual transmission.

It is crucial to this effort that we fight to make AIDS testing readily available and affordable in our schools. Testing is the only way a youngster can tell if she or her partner is infected. We have to take the politics and the stigma out of testing. Testing for HIV infection should be included in any physical examination when it is medically indicated. Your doctors should routinely test any patient for AIDS who has swollen glands, unexplained weight loss, fever, or any other problem that could indicate that he or she might have AIDS.

We can only put our future in the wide availability of testing, to identify infectious persons, together with promoting a sense of moral obligation to protect one's partners.

We desperately need drug rehabilitation programs and sex education programs that emphasize the *avoidance* of exposure to AIDS and the *elimination* of risks for women and adolescents *now!*

Some of the women of ancient Greece, yielding to their husbands' pressure and desiring sex themselves, found it difficult to say no. Lysistrata had to stop some who wanted to sneak home and make love. That would have sabotaged the peace strike. Lysistrata rallied the women and urged them to persist. She read them a "prophecy" which contained the following warning:

"But should these swallows, indulging their lust, lose heart, or dissolve their plots and singly depart, breaking the bands that bind them together, then know them as the worst birds that ever wore feathers." *

The language of this ancient Greek prose may seem a little strange to us, but Lysistrata's message is crystal clear: "Ladies, together we stand, divided we fall," a very timely message indeed!

If you are the only one in your crowd or at the office or in your community or in your town who says no to casual sex, the only one to make love within a mutually exclusive sexual relationship, the only one who limits sex to safe, dry practices unless she knows the man's AIDS status, if you are the oddball who inquires into her date's sexual and drug history, and if you are alone in insisting that he be tested before you go to bed with him, you will have a difficult battle.

If your daughter is the only one in her class, or at a party, or in her school, or on the block, who refuses to have sex with every date, who won't make love with a boy until they have a committed and sexually exclusive relationship, or who sticks to safe sex, she will have a tough time.

If the women who refuse to have sex until they are sure that their partners will not give them AIDS are not supported by other women, this is not going to work. If you're the only one who says no, the man will simply look for a more compliant woman.

But if men and boys find out that women are united in feeling entitled to protection, that *all* women expect men

* *Lysistrata*, Aristophanes, translated by Douglas Parker. A Mentor Book, 1964.

to behave responsibly and we *all* insist on making sure that a man is not infected before we will sleep with him, if he knows that he is just not going to get the kind of sex he wants unless he proves that he is not infected, then men's behavior will change. When the majority of women insist on safe sex or hold out on sex until she and her partner are ready to commit themselves to an exclusive relationship or marriage, when we stop "buying" the nonsense that asking him to wear a condom is healthy assertiveness, then men's behavior will change. Let us show them the way; they will eventually thank us!

Today in 1987 as I write this book fewer than one in ten thousand (0.01 percent) of our women are infected and only four in ten thousand (0.04 percent) men outside the high-risk groups. We are still essentially uncontaminated, but the growing number of the infected males who are having sex with women poses a great danger to women and children and ultimately for individuals everywhere.

The tidal wave has not yet hit us. But it is definitely on the horizon and coming at us at a terrific pace. If we close the bridge of women now we can still prevent a disaster.

We must help our young women to protect themselves by creating a social climate in which there is no stigma attached to AIDS testing, and where men will respect a woman's right to remain healthy, and where it is taken for granted that partners will not expose each other to AIDS.

We can not wait until the men stop their endless political wars and pass the right laws and until they put into effect public health policies that will protect women. These things may take forever and a day, and until this happens you simply have to take care of yourself, so that someday you will not have to admit to the man you love that you can't marry him or carry his baby, because you are carrying AIDS.

Op-Ed piece in *The New York Times*,
"The A.C.L.U.'s Myopic Stand on AIDS,"
by Charles Rembar, May 15, 1987.

The A.C.L.U.'s Myopic Stand on AIDS

BY CHARLES REMBAR *

Remarkably, the American Civil Liberties Union still adheres to a policy statement on AIDS that it issued in April 1986. The organization opposes testing for the AIDS virus unless a person wants it. It opposes reporting of cases of AIDS by doctors, hospitals and laboratories. It opposes tracing those with whom the harborer of the virus has had sexual contact. All in the name of privacy.

Though it may come as a surprise to most of its members, too often in important ways the A.C.L.U. is a conservative, backward-looking organization, trapped in vested doctrine. It clings to once useful concepts that are inappropriate to current problems. Like the French military, which prepared for World War II by building the Maginot Line, which was nicely adapted to the trench warfare of World War I, the A.C.L.U. sometimes hauls up legal arguments effective in old libertarian battles but irrelevant to those at hand.

For example, take literary censorship cases in the 1960's. In opposing censorship, the A.C.L.U. argued that publication of certain books created no "clear and present danger" to society. The "clear and present danger" argument, in the 1920's, had been used to protect from prosecution people who expressed political opinions without direct incitement to law-breaking. But

---

* Charles Rembar is a lawyer who has handled a number of constitutional law cases.

it had nothing to do with the question of whether and how far the First Amendment restricted anti-obscenity statutes.

Those who sought to suppress books they considered obscene did not argue that the books would cause an immediate conflagration. Rather, they had in mind the books' continuing effect on sexual morality. Censors presented the familiar slippery-slope argument: If the courts allowed the open publication of "Lady Chatterly's Lover," the next thing you know they would allow "Tropic of Cancer" and, after that, we would sink so low as to publish "Fanny Hill." (That, of course, is exactly what happened.)

Since the prospect of a gradual deterioration in morality over a period of time was put forward to justify suppression, it made no sense to argue that there was no *immediate and present* danger of instantaneous destruction of morality, as the A.C.L.U. did. Instead, the answer, as the Supreme Court held, was that a book that possessed some social value was part of the press, which the First Amendment guarded.

The A.C.L.U., again looking backward, today cannot depart from a concept of privacy that worked well for liberals in abortion cases heard by the courts. The nation — indeed, the world — faces the worst plague in history. The A.C.L.U., however, declares that efforts to deal with it are less important than the preservation of privacy. It finds no "compelling health purpose" in testing except at the option of an individual, in any requirement that test results showing the presence of the virus be identified and reported and in the tracing of sexual contacts.

In justifying these imperious pronouncements, the A.C.L.U. cites "basic constitutional guarantees," "individual rights" and "civil rights." These terms are far too vaporous to support a constitutional restriction on action by the states. A more concrete prohibition is required. The only one the A.C.L.U. cites is "the right to privacy."

There has been so much talk about privacy that it is worth recalling that the word "privacy" does not appear in the Constitution. The Supreme Court has, indeed, inferred a right of privacy in certain cases. But it carefully has limited its decisions to cases before it, and has explicitly denied that there exists any broad general right of privacy that can stand in the way of legislation important to the public welfare.

The Justices, or a majority of them, found a right of privacy in the First Amendment when someone was prosecuted for viewing pornographic material in his own home. They found it in the Fourth and Fifth Amendments when police behavior or other criminal enforcement tactics were too intrusive. They found it in the Bill of Rights generally when they sanctioned giving out birth control information. They found it in the 14th Amendment when they gave qualified approval to a personal choice on abortion. In these decisions, however, the Court took pains to make it clear that though a constitutional right of privacy exists in certain contexts, the right is "not unqualified." It is subject to a measure of "state regulation," and it must be weighed against "important state interests."

There is a difference of opinion in the medical profession about the danger of AIDS, but these differences all lie in a spectrum extending only from the terribly dangerous to the utterly disastrous. And no scientist sees any early development of a cure or vaccine.

In these circumstances, the situation we face falls well within the borders of the area in which the Court has said that the constitutional right of privacy must yield to considerations of public welfare. Attempts to limit the spread of the disease by compulsory testing, reporting and contact-tracing can reasonably be presumed to have some restraining effect on the travels of the virus.

One can advocate personal rights that go beyond the definitions the courts have given. Though the A.C.L.U. is basing its position on what it asserts are "constitutional guarantees," let us make it easier for the A.C.L.U. by shifting the issue from the law of privacy as it exists to the law as one might think it ought to be.

Is it good that there be testing that goes beyond an individual's request for it? Is it good that there be identification and reporting of those who carry the virus? Is it good that there be tracing of those to whom it may be reasonably supposed the virus has been transmitted and who may in turn transmit it to others?

Obviously these things are good. Are they, in the light of what we know about the disease, less important than privacy? The answer is plain, except to those so infatuated with personal rights as to ignore the sorest community needs.

Part of the horror of the disease is its certain outcome. The A.C.L.U., rather than receding from a cherished doctrine, would allow a number of people — perhaps a very large number — to die this horrid death. The organization apparently believes in a divine right of privacy, which reigns supreme above reason and common decency.

Letter to the staff of The New York Hospital advising us that the Health Department was still restricting HIV (AIDS) antibody testing as of March 17, 1987.

THE NEW YORK HOSPITAL
525 East Sixty-eighth Street
New York, N.Y., 10021
17 March 1987

Dear Doctor:

The Health Commissioners of NY, NJ and NYC, while stressing the current safety of blood transfusions and their low risk of AIDS, have said that patients or their families concerned about possible HIV infection due to prior transfusion should contact their physician or the hospital where they were transfused, and that anti-HIV testing is available for those desiring it.

The attached "Information for Physicians: Transmission of HIV by Transfusion," is provided by New York Blood Center for your use in dealing with patient inquiries about being tested. It explains how you can arrange for your patients to be tested and discusses special considerations such as the need for counseling and confidentiality.

Patients who contact New York Hospital in-patient services regarding previous transfusions and who seek HIV antibody testing may be referred to extension 4363 (472–4363) for further information and referral to a physician.

*HIV antibody testing is not currently performed by the Clinical Laboratories of The New York Hospital due to Health Department restrictions.** (An Information Bulletin will be issued when the restrictions are lifted.)

Meanwhile, if antibody testing is desired, the use of the State,

---

* Italics are mine to emphasize what I regard as inappropriate restriction or discouragement of AIDS antibody testing.

City, or New York Blood Center testing options for obtaining the HIV antibody test are suitable alternatives. These options are described in the attached materials (see enclosures). As soon as labels and forms for use of the latter option become available from the New York Blood Center, they will also be made available from the NYH Blood Bank on request for your convenience.

All blood transfused at The New York Hospital after April 9, 1985 (eight days prior to the NYBC date) was screened and found to be negative for HIV antibody.

Carl F.W. Wolf, M.D.
Director
Blood Bank & Transfusion
Service

Transcript of a phone conversation between a woman caller and the New York Health Department's "AIDS Hotline" which contains misinformation and inappropriate advice about condoms and AIDS testing for women, June 8, 1987. The asterisks mark misinformation and/or inappropriate advice.

AIDS Hotline: Hello.

Woman Caller: Hello.

AIDS Hotline: Wait a minute, will you hang on please?

WC: Sure.

AH: AIDS Hotline, can I help you?

WC: Yes, I want to inquire about testing, please.

AH: Sure. Um. Are you interested in taking the test?

WC: Yes. I want to take the test. I have already been exposed.

AH: Okay. Why do you think you are at risk?

WC: Well I had sex with a man who I think may be a bisexual.

AH: And how long ago was this?

WC: I would say about four weeks ago.

AH: Well, was it four weeks ago?

WC: Yes.

AH: And you have reason to believe he was bisexual?

WC: Yes.

AH: You have reason to believe he is infected?

WC: No. But that's a high-risk group, isn't it?

AH: Well, it depends. Not necessarily* — you don't have to worry about risk groups, you have to worry about behavior. Okay. Now is that someone you are still involved with?

WC: No.

AH: Okay, and he didn't use condoms.

WC: Yes he did.

AH: And did the condom break?

WC: No.

AH: Okay, and you had vaginal intercourse?

WC: Yes.

AH: Did you have anal intercourse?

WC: No.

AH: Okay, and did you have oral sex with him?

WC: No.

AH: And the condom didn't break?

WC: No.

AH: Then you're not at risk.* He didn't ejaculate into you?

WC: Well, that's not what it said on "Nightline."

AH: Did I speak to you earlier today?

WC: No.

AH: You didn't call here earlier today?

WC: No.

AH: Okay. Um, no, well that information . . . I don't know what exactly was said on "Nightline," but if a man is using condoms on you and he ejaculates and the condom hasn't broken then you can't get infected.*

WC: You can't?

AH: No, you can't. If the semen does not have any contact with your blood at all.

WC: Is that the only way you can get it? What about the moisture?

AH: No, not moisture. You have to worry about semen.

WC: I see. Boy, that . . . certainly the *Post* didn't say that but you know . . .

AH: Well, the *Post* is a rag . . .

WC: Yes?

AH: You should stop reading the *Post*. If you want to stay informed.

WC: Yes.

AH: I know that it's so anxiety-provoking.

WC: Yeah, it sure is. In other words, it's okay for me to sleep with my husband again, I can't infect him?

AH: No.* The chances . . . well, well . . . you . . . no that's fine . . . umm . . . female-to-male transmission is very low. There have only been four to five cases of women transmitting the virus.

WC: You know, that is so confusing. You hear in Africa it is fifty/fifty. Is that wrong?

AH: Well . . . yeah . . . The epidemiology of the disease in Africa is different from here.

WC: You mean in Africa women give it to men and here they don't?

AH: Well, I'm not sure about that. But in the United States in the cases we've studied there have only been four or five cases of men contracting the virus.

WC: I see. Well, that makes me feel better.

AH: Yeah, now . . .

WC: Now I also might be pregnant. I don't know yet.

AH: From this man. Well, that's not . . .

WC: No, no, no, no. Not from this man, from my husband.

AH: Oh, okay. Well, that's fine. Is your husband an IV drug user?

WC: No, no, no, I'm only worried about this man because I heard there's a big failure rate with condoms even if they don't break.

AH: As long as the condom didn't break . . .

WC: Uh huh . . .

AH: You're fine. There's no problem.*

WC: Uh huh . . . and you don't advise testing and you don't think I have to worry about my baby or about my husband . . .

AH: No.*

WC: Okay. Well . . .

AH: No . . .

WC: What if I'm nervous anyway, I think, I'm nervous, anyway, because you hear different stories, you know.

AH: Well, do you have a, um, do you see a therapist?

WC: No. I'm not a nervous person.

AH: Well, people see therapists for many reasons.

WC: I don't have any reasons to see a therapist.

AH: I think the best thing that you should do . . .

WC: Yes?

AH: . . . is to keep yourself informed.

WC: Yes . . .

AH: Buy *The New York Times*, the AIDS articles are in the *Times* regularly.

WC: Well, the *Times* said there was a study in Miami where they showed a big failure rate in heterosexual transmission.

AH: A failure rate of what? Condoms?

WC: Yeah . . . without breaking . . . down in Miami University . . . that's where I got nervous first . . .

AH: Um hmm . . . well, you know there are all sorts of different research going on.

WC: Uh huh . . .

AH: All over the world. However, if a condom is used properly and doesn't break, that semen has never had any contact with your blood.*

WC: But it said that you can also get it from saliva . . .

AH: There hasn't been one case of anyone contracting the virus from saliva.

WC: Ah huh . . . ah huh . . .

AH: Now if someone's infected . . .

WC: Yes . . .

AH: The HIV virus, the antibodies are present in their saliva . . .

WC: Oh, I thought it was the infected cell, not the antibody.

AH: No, it's the antibodies that are present in the saliva of an infected individual. Okay.*

WC: Uh huh . . .

AH: However, there hasn't been a case . . .

WC: I see.

AH: . . . of anyone contracting it. We would still advise you not to . . .

WC: Well, I'm not in that position . . . I'm just confused because *The New York Times* says there is a danger with condoms even if they don't break and the health department says not. So I may be having a baby, you can understand why I'd be a little frightened.

AH: Right. Do you have a regular gynecologist?

WC: Yes.

AH: Okay, can you talk to her about these things?

WC: It's a he . . .

AH: Oh.

WC: . . . and he suggested I be tested because he said you can even get it through breast milk.

AH: But, whose breast milk have you been having? *

WC: No . . . no . . . if I'm infected by this guy and I have a baby, even the baby can get it from the breast milk. That's what my gynecologist at New York Hospital says.

AH: Okay. And how long . . . you had . . . uh . . . you slept with this man a month ago . . .

WC: Four weeks ago.

AH: Four weeks ago.

WC: Yes, four weeks ago.

AH: Okay . . . um . . . you would need to wait five more months.

WC: Oh really?

AH: Before being tested.

WC: Five months . . .

AH: Because the antibodies if you were exposed might not appear in your blood for six months.

WC: But gee, that . . . see how crazy once again . . . My gynecologist says that between two and six weeks most people show up with antibodies and you should be tested at six months again.

AH: Yeah, but most people will . . . but what happens if you have been exposed, you take the test too soon. You test negative, but in fact had you waited a proper amount of time . . .

WC: But why don't you just retest then . . .

AH: Well, how many times are you going to take the test?

WC: Twice. That's what he said.

AH: Well, what's the point of that?

WC: Because . . .

AH: He makes more money and . . .*

WC: No, no, no . . . I thought this is free from the health department.

AH: Well, there are city tests that are free . . .

WC: Yeah, so why can't you take it twice?

AH: Well, that's wasteful, isn't it?* Don't you think?

WC: Well, not really, because he said there's a 90 percent chance if after six weeks you're negative you're okay, but just to make sure you should take it again in six months.

AH: Well, the idea is we advise you to take the test just once and we won't schedule you for an appointment here unless you waited an adequate amount of time.

WC: Until I waited six months you won't schedule me.

AH: Right. Because this way you'll know that your test is all right.

WC: And what do you tell people to do in the meanwhile? You know, I have . . .

AH: We tell them to practice safe sex.

WC: Which is? What's safe?

AH: What's safe? Have you ever heard of safe sex?

WC: Well, I hear three different stories. One says you should only be monogamous. That's the only safe thing to do. That's what . . . you know . . . that's what I hear. Is that true?

AH: Well, you have to understand that you have to make certain choices for yourself . . .

WC: Sure . . .

AH: If you want to be monogamous, that's your choice.

WC: But is that safe?

AH: Well, what if you're monogamous with someone who's infected and he's not using a condom. Is that safe?

WC: So you think I should have my husband tested and make sure he's safe?

AH: No, I didn't say you should . . . You told me you had nothing to worry about with your husband.* Is your husband an IV drug user?

WC: No.

AH: And he's not having sex with other men?

WC: No.

AH: Okay, what are you worried about?

WC: But it is safe to be monogamous?

AH: Sure, if you're with someone you don't think is infected and if they are infected that they are using a condom.*

WC: And you mean condoms make it safe?

AH: Yes, if you have sex with a man and he uses a condom and it doesn't break and semen does not enter your bloodstream then . . .*

WC: That has been shown scientifically?

AH: Hm Hmmm.

WC: Will you just give me one reference to that article because I want to show my gynecologist because that is the opposite of what he told me, so I'd love to tell him what the health department is advising.

AH: Okay. I'm going to put you on hold. Hold on.

WC: Sure.

A directive restricting AIDS testing sent to physicians by the New York City Health Department in 1985.

THE CITY OF NEW YORK
DEPARTMENT OF HEALTH
125 WORTH ST., NEW YORK, N.Y. 10013

Dear Colleague:

The New York City Department of Health is offering HTLV-III antibody testing as part of a research protocol designed to better evaluate the characteristics of commercially available HTLV-III testing kits. The use of HTLV-III antibody testing kits by commercial laboratories, except for blood banking purposes or as part of an identified research protocol, *has been restricted by the Commissioner of Health* * (see attached regulation). Testing will be available to persons only through licensed physicians. Persons being tested will have read an information statement on HTLV-III antibody testing and signed informed consent. The confidentiality of participant's will be protected — only the physician will have the participant's name. There will be *a delay of notification of test results* * of weeks to several months in order to assure laboratory accuracy of test results.

Attached is the Department of Health's protocol which includes important information statements on HTLV-III testing, consent forms, specimen submission forms, physicians' instructions and the Commissioner's regulation on HTLV-III testing. The consent forms, important information statements on HTLV-III, and specimen submission forms may be duplicated.

* Italics throughout Appendix D are mine to emphasize what I regard as inappropriate restriction or discouragement of AIDS antibody testing.

If you have questions, or need more materials, please telephone 1-718-HTLV-111.

Sincerely,
Rand Stonebaner, M.D.
Director,
AIDS Program

PROTOCOL FOR DEVELOPMENT OF QUALITY CONTROL FOR ANTI-HTLV-III ANTIBODY TESTING NEW YORK CITY DEPARTMENT OF HEALTH

INTRODUCTION:

The imminent release of serological testing kits for HTLV-III, a retrovirus which is a suspected cause of AIDS, is a serious social and public health challenge for the New York City Department of Health. Little data have been released, to date, on the characteristics of these tests (sensitivity and specificity), and their value for general screening is unknown (predictive value). Further, the interpretation of a positive test is unclear: thus, for individuals a positive test result may cause unnecessary psychological harm, as well as unjustified social discrimination. The purpose of this proposal is to better evaluate the characteristics of commercially-available HTLV-III testing kits, particularly related to their use in healthy populations with low prevalence of disease.

STUDY DESIGN:

Sera from participants in this research will be from two sources: the first will be samples of sera testing positive and negative on ELISA-screening from the New York Blood Center; the second will be from any NYC physicians who wish to cooperate in the study by submitting samples under strict confidentiality and study protocol. Physicians will also include information about age, sex, health and AIDS risk group status of the participant on the specimen submission form. Before study entry, a participant must read an information statement on HTLV-III antibody testing and give informed consent. This research will proceed as several concurrent experiments, as follows:

1. *Comparability of 5 manufacturer's test kits:*
   A portion of available specimens will be tested on all 5 kits. Agreement will be assessed by a multiple correlation coefficient or alpha-coefficient, which measures agreement across independent tests. Patterns of agreement among groups of tests will be described.

2. *Reliability of 5 manufacturer's test kits:*
   A portion of available specimens will be tested twice on each type of test kit. Reliability coefficients and a variant of the kappa-statistic will be used to evaluate the reproducibility of test kits.

3. *Evaluation of test kits when a-priori probability of positivity is very high or very low:*
   Serum specimens submitted in cooperation with the New York Blood Center which tested initially positive or negative on a single ELISA test procedure will be subjected to the designs (1) and (2) above. The performance of tests varies markedly by prevalence of true positives in test samples: this allows us to evaluate all 5 manufacturer's kits at extremes of expected population prevalence of true positives. We will be able to estimate predictive value of a positive test given various prevalences of true positives.

4. *Comparability of ELISA with other methods:*
   A sample of ELISA positives, negatives and undetermined sera from (1) and (2) above will be further tested with the Western Blot method.

5. *Statistical analysis of cutpoints for defining positive and negative test results, to maximize test sensitivity and specificity:*
   ELISA test results are read as optical densities, on a continuous logarithmic scale. The distribution of each manufacturer's test results on positive and negative sera will be examined. Adjustment of cutpoints to maximize sensitivity and specificity will be explored.

Data analysis will be completed using the City of New York's Computer Service Center's facilities. There will be careful restriction of access to all data until analyses are thorough and complete.

LABORATORY METHODS
1. ELISA

2. Western Blot
3. T-cell Phenotyping

Test results will be sent to the submitting physicians after repro-ducibility of the test has been demonstrated. This will impose an initial delay of one to several months between submission and result, which may decrease after the beginning of the study. Some individuals will be re-contacted through their physicians for repeat testing at a later date. Specimens will be received at the Bureau of Labs, 455 First Avenue 24 hours/day. Specimens must be received within 24–48 hours after collection.

INFORMED CONSENT
Written informed consent will be obtained from each participant by the enrolling physician. The voluntary nature of participa-tion, potential risks and benefits to the patient and the intended use of the clinical specimens will be explained in full. An impor-tant information statement about HTLV-III antibody testing and its significance to the participant will be included in the consent. The physician will be responsible for keeping the original in-formed consent.

CONFIDENTIALITY AND RECORD MANAGEMENT
The confidentiality of participants will be protected by the New York City Department of Health. The name and identification of each participant will only be known by the physician whom the participant has contacted in order to enroll in the study. The *participant's* physician will assign an identification code to the participant based on the physician's 3 initials and a numerical code of 001 to 999 for each participant enrolled from a particular physician. Physicians will be responsible for maintaining records on each participant so, if need be, the participant could be con-tacted by the physician if the NYCDOH requests further blood specimens for retesting.

NYCDOH HTLV-III ANTIBODY TESTING STUDY INSTRUCTIONS TO PHYSICIANS

1. The consent and the form entitled "Important Information About HTLV-III Antibody Testing" must be read and signed by the participant in the presence of a witness. No alteration to the consent document may be made.
2. Blood collection procedure:

   A. *for HTLV-III antibody testing* 10cc of blood must be collected in an evacuated tube without anticoagulant (red top tube) and received by the Bureau of Labs within 24–48 hours.
   B. all specimens must be labeled with the following:
      1. date and time of specimen collection.
      2. specimen code, consisting of physician's three initials plus a numerical code from 001 to 999 for the patient's identification
         example: second patient of Dr. John D. Smith, code "JDS002"
         Note — Physician is responsible for maintaining patient code records.
      3. if a second specimen is requested on a patient enter same code and specify second or third draw etc.
   C. all specimens must be received with the Specimen Submission Form and Memorandum of Understanding statement signed by the physician.
   D. specimens are to be delivered to the New York City Bureau of Laboratories, 455 First Avenue, New York, NY, which is open 24 hours a day.
   E. For further information call the HTLV Hotline at 1-718-HTLV-111.

NEW YORK CITY DEPARTMENT OF HEALTH HTLV-III ANTIBODY PROFICIENCY TESTING PROTOCOL CONSENT FORM FOR SPECIMEN COLLECTION

The New York City Department of Health (NYCDOH) is offering HTLV-III antibody testing as a part of an epidemiologic investigation which will help us better understand what the test means. HTLV-III antibody testing for a limited period of time will only be performed by the NYCDOH, and the test will only be available through your physician. The use of HTLV-III antibody testing by labs other than those involved in screening of the blood supply or (organ donors) is *currently restricted by the Department of Health.* * If you and your physician agree that performing the HTLV-III antibody test on you is in your best interest, you should be aware of the following: knowledge is limited about what a positive test means; that there *exists a possibility that a positive test result could cause unnecessary psychological stress for you; and that their exists a potential that positive test results could be used to discriminate against you if they were not kept confidential.*

This study is designed to compare the results of commercially available HTLV-III antibody tests which use the enzyme-linked immunosorbent assay (ELISA) method in order to assure reliability of results and quality control. Your blood will be tested by at least two ELISA methods and may be further tested by another method to detect antibody (Western Blot). Your T-cells (a type of white blood cell) will also be measured in order to determine what relationship their numbers have to your HTLV-III antibody results. The results of the HTLV-III antibody test will not be released to your physician until we are certain of the quality of our testing methods, which could take several weeks.

If you agree to participate in this investigation, your physician will collect 1¼ tablespoons of blood for antibody testing and T-cell studies. You may be contacted through your physician for a second specimen for further testing. When the blood sample is taken, you may have some slight discomfort at the site of entry of the needle, and a small bruise may develop. Otherwise there is no likely risk of physical injury.

If you do not wish to participate in this study, it will not affect any treatment or services that you may be currenty receiving, or that in the future you may be entitled to receive, from the New York City Department of Health or _____.

(Physician or Hospital)

Your physician will also be requested to submit with your specimen certain information about you regarding your present health, as well as whether or not you may be in a group at high risk to develop AIDS (i.e., homosexual male, I.V. drug user, blood product recipient, or sexual partner of any of these groups).

All of the information obtained about you is absolutely confidential. Only your doctor will know your name, or other identifying information. The New York City Department of Health will receive an identification code assigned to you by your physician on the submitted specimens. Reports of your HTLV-III antibody results or requests for further specimen submission from you will be communicated using this assigned code to your physician.

The information gained from this investigation will help contribute toward learning about the meaning of the results of currently available HTLV-III antibody tests. There is no guarantee that you will personally benefit by participating in this study.

I have read and understand the preceding information as well as the important information statement about HTLV-III antibody testing which I have signed unaltered. I realize the limitations and risks of HTLV-III antibody testing based on current knowledge. Any questions I had have been answered satisfactorily. I have discussed the confidentiality of my HTLV-III antibody results with respect to my medical records with my physician. If I have further questions, I understand I may contact the Department of Health's HTLV-III Hotline at 1-718-HTLV-111, or my physician.

_____   _____
Signature of Physician or,   Signature of Participant
Physician staff member

                                 __ __ / __ __ / __ __
                                         Date

IMPORTANT INFORMATION STATEMENT ON HTLV-III ANTIBODY TESTING

It is extremely important that you read and understand the following about HTLV-III Antibody Testing

A virus, now known as HTLV-III (human T-lymphotropic virus-type III) or LAV (lymphadenopathy-associated virus), is associated with AIDS (acquired immunodeficiency syndrome) and is probably the cause. Antibody tests to detect exposure to HTLV-III have been developed recently and are now available. This test is licensed solely for the purpose of screening donated blood, in order to eliminate blood which may contain HTLV-III virus from the blood supply. However, the test may become available to you through other sources. It is important that anyone who desires to be tested for HTLV-III is aware of the following serious problems associated with the test.

- If you get a positive result nobody knows what this means regarding your future health.
- If your test result is not kept confidential you could be wrongly discriminated against.

Based on our present knowledge, a positive HTLV-III antibody test probably means that you have, in the past, been exposed to HTLV-III or a similar virus. However, it is unknown if a positive test means that:

- *You may have been infected in the past, have recovered, and are no longer infectious to others and will not become ill as a result of this exposure.*
- *You may be currently infected with HTLV-III virus and may be able to transmit it to others.*
- You may be currently infected and may develop AIDS or a related condition at some unknown time in the future.

Also, the test could be wrong. You may have never been exposed to the virus. This is a false positive and is always a small possibility with laboratory tests.

A negative test probably means that you have not been exposed to HTLV-III virus. But in some situations persons known to be infected with the virus also test negative. These are called false negatives.

Because of the limited knowledge about how to interpret a positive test, the HTLV-III antibody test is not:

- A test for AIDS
- A test to predict if you may later become ill with AIDS or a related condition
- A test to predict if you are protected (immune) from the AIDS-associated virus
- A test to determine if you may transmit the AIDS-associated virus to others.

Therefore, at this time there exists a real possibility that a positive test may be harmful to you in several ways.

14   The *New York Times* editorial objecting to AIDS testing on erroneous grounds, "When to Test for AIDS," May 17, 1987.

When to Test for AIDS

Why not compel everyone to be tested for AIDS as the basis for halting further spread of the virus? That's a natural first thought to anyone who ponders the deadly epidemic. But it's only a first thought. That some senior Administration officials argue for mandatory AIDS testing shows how late in the day they have arrived at step one.

William Bennett, the Secretary of Education, wants AIDS tests to be given to everyone admitted to the hospital or applying for a marriage license. Gary Bauer, a senior White House aide, says opponents of such tests are promoting "a bizarre type of enforced ignorance." The Public Health Service now says that all immigrants will be screened for AIDS virus.

There are at least six reasons for believing that advocates of general forced testing are opinionated, hasty or poorly informed.

Lesson One: Don't drive victims underground. Homosexuals and intravenous drug abusers, the principal victims, are not mainstream America. Living at the edge of social tolerance in many states, they face plenty of discrimination already. Their cooperation in changing their own behavior is crucial in slowing the disease's spread to other groups. Mandatory testing is the surest way to discourage them from contact with health authorities.

Lesson Two: A consensus is not a conspiracy. No one should lightly deny public health officials the tools they need to combat AIDS, including use of the AIDS antibody tests. What public officials want — for the reason cited above — is more voluntary testing, not mandatory testing. Mr. Bennett seems to believe that the Federal public health agency has fallen under the influence of homosexuals who oppose mandatory testing for self-interested reasons. But the reason for agreement is not conspiracy. Both groups believe voluntary testing is the better way of halting AIDS.

Lesson Three: Why in hospitals? Hospital patients are predominantly the elderly and the very young, two categories least likely to have AIDS. Why does Mr. Bennett propose to look there for the virus instead of among high-risk groups? Because hospitals are where testing is easiest. So too argued the drunkard who lost his keys 'in the dark and explained he was searching for them under the lamp post because the light was better.

Lesson Four: Like it or not, morals have changed. Many states require a syphilis test for those seeking a marriage license. Mr. Bennett can't understand why an AIDS test isn't given too. The reason is that a minute proportion of known syphilis cases are detected this way. New York recently dropped the syphilis test because the results were not worth the cost, and because of suspicion that some couples nowadays have sex before marriage. The same logic applies to AIDS, but there's another more cogent reason.

*Lesson Five: False alarms have grim consequences.** The two present tests for AIDS virus are highly specific but even in conjunction are not totally accurate. The danger of "false positives" — diagnosing individuals as exposed to AIDS when they are not — is probably minuscule with high-risk populations. But the danger grows rapidly when screening large populations at low risk.

According to a paper to be published shortly by Michael J. Barry and colleagues at the Harvard School of Public Health, the two standard AIDS tests would identify 28 true positives, 2 false negatives and 11 false positives when applied to a low-risk population, defined as 30 AIDS cases, per 100,000 people. What those figures say is that, for every 28 cases correctly diagnosed, the tests risk falsely informing 11 individuals that they carry the virus of a deadly disease and should never have children. Without guarantees of confidentiality, the insurers, employers, landlords and classmates of these 11 individuals may also learn, and act, on the false information. What a burden for mandatory testers to bear.

* Boxed material, in my opinion, inappropriately discourages AIDS antibody testing.

Lesson Six: AIDS makes a poor political football. Mr. Bauer believes that public health officials have few qualms in urging explicit sex education for young children, offensive as that may be to conservatives. But when it comes to testing, "the left's political agenda takes over." He says, "Either this is potentially the Black Death or it isn't." In fact, no one knows how widely AIDS will spread, but it's prudent to take precautions. Teaching teen-agers safe sex is an effective precaution — and mandatory testing is not.

AIDS is a medical issue. Those who politicize it, or see political motives where none exist, are seriously delaying national policy on AIDS and measures to save lives. The only known way to curb AIDS is to persuade people to change behavior. The Administration still has not mounted a massive public education program of the sort already under way at several European countries. The Secretary of Education should be leading the charge for education about AIDS and voluntary testing. Mandatory testing should be his last thought, not his first.

Op-Ed piece in *The New York Times*,
"On AIDS and Moral Duty,"
by Willard Gaylin, M.D., April 24, 1987.

On AIDS and Moral Duty

BY WILLARD GAYLIN *

BRIARCLIFF MANOR, N.Y. — Potential AIDS victims who refuse to be tested for the disease and then defend their right to remain ignorant about whether they carry the virus are entitled to that right. But ignorance cannot be used to rationalize irresponsibility. Nowhere in their argument is there concern about how such ignorance might endanger public health by exposing others to the virus.

All disease is an outrage, and disease that affects the young and healthy seems particularly outrageous. When a disease selectively attacks the socially disadvantaged such as homosexuals and drug abusers, it seems an injustice beyond rationalization. Such is the case with acquired immune deficiency syndrome.

Decent people are offended by this unfairness and in the name of benevolence have been driven to do morally irresponsible things such as denying the unpleasant facts of the disease, out of compassion for the victims. We cannot fudge the facts to comfort the afflicted when such obfuscation compounds the tragedy.

Some crucial facts: AIDS is a communicable disease. The percentage of those infected with the AIDS virus who will eventually contract the disease is unknown, but that percentage rises with each new estimate. The disease so far has been 100 percent fatal. The latency period between the time the virus is acquired and the disease develops is also unknown.

We now have tests for the presence of the virus that are as efficient and reliable as almost any diagnostic test in medicine. An individual who tests positive can be presumed with near-certainty to carry the virus, whether he has the disease or not.

* Willard Gaylin is president of the Hastings Center, a public-policy organization.

To state that the test for AIDS is "ambiguous," as a clergyman recently said in public, is a misstatement and an immoral act. To state that the test does not directly indicate the presence of the virus is a half truth that misleads and an immoral act. The test correlates so consistently with the presence of the virus in bacteria cultures as to be considered 100 percent certain by experts.

Everyone who tests positive must understand that he is a potential vector for the AIDS virus and has a moral duty and responsibility to protect others from contamination. We need not force everyone in high-risk populations to take the test. There is no treatment for the disease. Therefore, to insist on testing serves no therapeutic purpose.

Certainly there are those who would prefer ambiguity to certitude. However, a person who is at risk and refuses to have himself tested must behave as though he had been tested and found positive. To do otherwise is cowardice compounding hypocrisy with wrongdoing.

Surely an individual has a right to spare himself the agony of knowledge if he prefers wishful thinking to certitude. He must not use his desire for hope as an excuse for denial.

We have a duty to protect the innocent and the unborn. Voluntary premarital testing for AIDS is a protection for both partners and for the uncontaminated and unborn children. We know that AIDS is transmissible from male to female, from female to male, from parent to conceived child. We are dealing not just with the protection of the innocent but with an essential step to contain the spread of an epidemic as tragic and as horrible as any that has befallen modern man. We must do everything in our power to keep this still untreatable disease from becoming pandemic.

It may seem unfair to burden the tragic victims with concern for the welfare of others. But moral responsibility is not a luxury of the fortunate, and evil actions perpetrated in despair cannot be condoned out of pity. It is morally wrong for a healthy individual who tests positive for AIDS to be involved with anyone except under the strictest precautions now defined as safe sex.

It is morally wrong for someone in a high risk population who refuses to test himself to do other than to assume that he tests positively. It is morally wrong for those who, out of sympathy for the heartbreaking victims of this epidemic, act as though well-wishing and platitudes about the ambiguities of the disease are necessary in order to comfort the victims while they contribute to enlarging the number of those victims. Moral responsibility is the burden of the sick as well as the healthy.

Letter to *The New York Times* by Michael Marmor correcting Mr. Barnes, "Second AIDS Tests Increase Accuracy Dramatically," May 23, 1987.

Second AIDS Tests Increase Accuracy Dramatically

To the Editor:

Your May 5 letter from Mark Barnes, "AIDS Test Is, Unfortunately, Still Ambiguous," gave the misleading impression that current blood tests for antibodies to HIV, the human immunodeficiency virus that causes acquired immune deficiency syndrome, are inaccurate. In that this idea could discourage testing, it might have lethal consequences.

Mr. Barnes stated that the enzyme-linked immunosorbent assay, or ELISA, which is used to detect antibodies that signify exposure to HIV, is inaccurate when applied to populations with low rates of HIV infection. In this he is correct.

Even an accurate test that produces a low rate of "false positives" will be inaccurate when applied to populations containing few "true positives." Suppose, for example, that the ELISA has a false positive rate of .18 percent. Then, if 10,000 New York City adults were tested whose only risk for AIDS was heterosexual sex, and 10 were truly infected with HIV, the false positive rate of .18 percent would have to be applied to 9,990 uninfected persons.

As a result, 18 of these uninfected people (.0018 times 9,990) would be declared antibody-positive, or infected. Only 10 out of 28 total positives (10 true positives, plus 18 false positives), or 36 percent of the positives, truly would be infected. A positive result thus could not be given much credence.

However, all responsible testing laboratories are using a second, confirmatory test whenever a positive result occurs on the ELISA. By retesting positive samples with the Western blot test or some other confirmatory test, almost all false positive results are eliminated, while true positives are retained.

The accuracy of the two combined tests is very close to 100 percent, even in a low-prevalence population, even though either test used alone would be inaccurate in such a population.

In high-prevalence populations, such as homosexual men or intravenous drug users in New York City, the ELISA alone would be quite accurate. The technique of stringing two tests together, known as serial testing, is a well-known device commonly used in public health to address the problem of testing low-prevalence populations.

The expense of Western blot testing is not, as Mr. Barnes stated, prohibitive, because the test is used only on samples that are positive on the ELISA.

The HIV antibody tests and education concerning how the virus is spread are the only tools we have right now to contain the AIDS epidemic. People who are positive on blood testing must be assumed to be capable of infecting others. People who take the test and find they are infected can take precautions to avoid infecting their partners in sex or drug abuse, and to avoid bearing infected offspring. Individual test results can personalize moral responsibilities during the AIDS epidemic in ways that mass education cannot.

Incorrect information on the accuracy of HIV blood testing is potentially damaging to public health. The ultimate toll extracted by AIDS will be increased by statements that incorrectly discourage the use of the HIV blood tests.

Michael Marmor
Associate Professor
N.Y.U. Medical Center
New York, May 8, 1987

_____ APPENDIX H

Letter advising the staff of The New York Hospital about blood transfusions and AIDS risk, July 17, 1986.

THE NEW YORK HOSPITAL
Informational Bulletin #43–86
July 17, 1986

TO: Administrative Department Heads
Clinical Department Heads
Nursing Service
Unit Administration
Attending and Courtesy Staff
Graduate Staff
Cornell University Medical College

SUBJECT: Blood Transfusion and AIDS Risk

Sensational media reports about the safety of blood transfused to patients in our region have caused considerable patient anxiety. The reports were triggered by plans of blood collection agencies to notify those who received blood transfusion from prior donations by persons who were later found positive for antibody to HIV (HTLV-III). The following information is presented to place the true risks implied by the reports into perspective.

It is anticipated that, from 1977–1986, of the more than 2.7 million patients who received blood from the NYBC, about 700 persons will be notified of possible exposure to the HTLV-III virus. Because the rate of infection in donors was lower earlier in the epidemic, only $\frac{1}{3}$ to $\frac{1}{2}$ may actually have been infected. For persons who received transfusions in the past, their individual risk of having been infected is estimated at about 1 in 10,000.

Patients who received transfusions may approach their physicians to discuss whether it would be appropriate for them to be tested for HTLV-III antibody, an assay available through public health agencies.

Overall, an estimated 30% of infected individuals will develop AIDS after 6 to 8 years. Hemophiliacs appear to be different and about 1% have so far developed the disease. Transfusion recipients may therefore also exhibit a lower rate of disease after infection.

With respect to blood supply safety at the present time, the risk of a "false negative" donor test on current donations for transfusion *is about 1 in 250,000*. Therefore, of the 330,000 recipients of transfusions in the greater metropolitan region each year, it is highly unlikely now that more than one person might be exposed to the virus. This rate is similar to that for being hit by lightning in the U.S.

The chance of a patient having been exposed in the past is very small. The chance of a patient being exposed now is so small that public health officials now consider the blood supply as safe or safer than it has ever been.

Source: Press Conference, NY Blood Center, 7/16/86.

David D. Thompson, M.D.
Director

Scientific and Technical References

I. *The Epidemiology of AIDS*
1. Centers for Disease Control, "Update on Acquired Immune Deficiency Syndrome (AIDS) Among Patients With Hemophilia." *Morbidity and Mortality Weekly Reports*, 1982.
2. Centers for Disease Control, "Possible Transfusion-Associated Acquired Immunodeficiency Syndrome (AIDS): California." *Morbidity and Mortality Weekly Reports*, 1982.
3. Piot, P., et al., "Acquired Immunodeficiency Syndrome in a Heterosexual Population in Zaire." *Lancet*, 1984.
4. Brun-Vezinet, F., et al., "Prevelance of Antibodies to LAV in African Patients with AIDS." *Science*, 1985.
5. Jaffe, J.W., et al., "The Acquired Immunodeficiency Syndrome in Gay Men." *Annals of Internal Medicine*, 1985.
6. Blatter, W.A., et al., "Epidemiology of Human T-Lymphotropic Virus Type III and the Risk of AIDS." *Annals of Internal Medicine*, 1985.
7. Centers for Disease Control, "Update: Acquired Immunodeficiency Syndrome (AIDS) in the United States." *Morbidity and Mortality Weekly Reports*, 1986.
8. Redfield, R.R., and Burke, D.S., "Shadow on the Land: The Epidemiology of HIV Infection." *American Journal of Immunology*, 1987.
9. Burke, D.F., Brundage, J.F., and Bernier, W., "Demography of HIV Infections Among Military Recruit Applicants in New York City." *New York State Journal of Medicine*, May 1987.
10. Imperato, P.J., "Acquired Immunodeficiency Syndrome — 1987." *New York State Journal of Medicine*, May 1987.
11. Drucker, E., "AIDS: The Eleventh Year." *New York State Journal of Medicine*, May 1987.
12. Arno, P.S., and Hughes, R.G., "Local Policy Response to the AIDS Epidemic." *New York State Journal of Medicine*, May 1987.
13. Echenberg, D.F., "Education and Contact Notification for AIDS Prevention." *New York State Journal of Medicine*, May 1987.
14. Guinan, M.E., and Hardy, A., "Epidemiology of AIDS in Women in the United States." *Journal of the American Medical Association*, 1987.
15. Winkelstein, W., et al., "Sexual Practices and Risks of Infec-

tion by HIV." *Journal of the American Medical Association*, 1987.

16. Centers for Disease Control, *AIDS Surveillance Update*, April 29, 1987.

17. *Focus on AIDS, Symposium Proceedings*, under an educational grant from the Mérieux Institute, Inc., October 8, 1984.

18. "Report on AIDS in Cuba." *Garina* (a Havana, Cuba, newspaper), April 17, 1987.

19. Schorr, J.B., et al., "Prevalence of HLTV-III Antibody in American Blood Donors." *New England Journal of Medicine*, 1985.

20. Slivak, S.L., and Wormser, G.P., "How Common Is HTLV-III Infection in the U.S.?" *New England Journal of Medicine*, 1985.

21. Centers for Disease Control, "Antibody Prevalence in U.S. Military Applicants." *Morbidity and Mortality Weekly Reports*, 1986.

22. Centers for Disease Control, "Trends in HIV Infection Among Civilian Applicants for Military Service in the United States, October 1985–December 1986." *Morbidity and Mortality Weekly Reports*, 1987.

23. Fauci, A.S., "AIDS—Pathogenic Mechanisms and Research Strategies." *American Society for Microbiology News*, 1987.

24. Fauci, A.S., and Lane, C.: "Acquired Immunodeficiency Syndrome (AIDS)." In Harrison's *Principles of Internal Medicine, 11th Edition*; Braunwald, et. al. Ed., McGraw Hill, N.Y., 1987.

25. Norwood, C., *Advice for Life: A Woman's Guide to AIDS Risks and Prevention*. Pantheon, N.Y., 1987.

II. *Aids in Children and the Transmission of the HIV from Infected Mothers to Their Babies During Pregnancy*

1. Rubinstein, A., et al., "Acquired Immunodeficiency with Reversed T4/T8 Ratios in Infants Born to Promiscuous and Drug-Addicted Mothers." *Journal of the American Medical Association*, 1983.

2. Joviasas, E., et al., "LAV/HTLV-III in 20-Week Fetus." *Lancet*, 1985.

3. Scott, G.B., et al., "Mothers of Infants with the Acquired Immunodeficiency Syndrome: Evidence for Both Symptomatic and Asymptomatic Carriers." *Journal of the American Medical Association*, 1985.

4. Centers for Disease Control, "Recommendations for Assisting in the Prevention of Acquired Immunodeficiency Syndrome." *Morbidity and Mortality Weekly Reports*, 1985.
5. Pinching, A.J., and Jeffries, D.J., "AIDS and HTLV-III/LAV Infection: Consequences for Obstetrics and Perinatal Medicine." *British Journal of Obstetrics and Gynecology*, 1985.
6. Rubinstein, A., and Bernstein, L., "The Epidemiology of Pediatric Acquired Immunodeficiency Syndrome." *Clinical Immunology and Immunopathology*, 1986.
7. Centers for Disease Control, "Classification System for HIV Infection in Children Under 13 Years of Age." *Morbidity and Mortality Weekly Reports*, 1987.
8. Hein, K., "AIDS in Adolescents: A Rationale for Concern." *New York State Journal of Medicine*, May 1987.
9. Oxtoby, M.J., et al., "National Trends in Perinatally Acquired AIDS: United States. *III International Conference on AIDS*, Washington, D.C., June 1987.
10. Willoughby, A., et al., "Human Immunodeficiency in Pregnant Women and Their Offspring." *III International Conference on AIDS*, Washington, D.C., June 1987.

III. *Condoms*

1. Von Doring, G.K., "Is Das Kondom Heute Besser Als Sein Ruf?" (Is Today's Condom Better Than Its Reputation?) *Fortschritte Der Medicine*, 1980.
2. Hicks, D.R., et al., "Inactivation of HTLV/LAV-Infected Cultures of Normal Human Lymphocytes by Nonoxynol-9." *Lancet*, 1985.
3. Conant, M., et al., "Condoms Prevent the Transmission of AIDS-Associated Retrovirus." *Journal of the American Medical Association*, 1986.
4. Sophocles, A.M., and Brozovich, "Birth Control Failures Among Patients with Unwanted Pregnancies: 1982–1984." *Journal of Family Practice*, 1986.
5. Grady, W.R., et al., "Contraceptive Failures in the United States: National Survey of Family Growth." *Family Planning Perspectives*, 1986.
6. Fischl, M.A., Dickinson, G.W., et al., "Evaluation of Heterosexual Partners, Children, and Household Contacts of Adults with AIDS." *Journal of the American Medical Association*, February 1987.
7. Goldert, J.J., "What Is Safe Sex?" *New England Journal of Medicine*, 1987.

IV. *The AIDS Tests, Counseling, and Prevention*
  1. Weiss, S.H.; Goedert, J.J.; et al., "Screening Test for HTLV-III (AIDS Agent) Antibodies: Specificity, Sensitivity, and Applications." *Journal of the American Medical Association,* 1985.
  2. Biggar, R.J.; Gigase, P.L.; et al., "ELISA HTLV Retrovirus Antibody Reactivity Associated with Malaria and Immune Complexes in Healthy Africans." *Lancet,* 1985.
  3. Prentice, R.L.; Collins; R.J.; et. al., "Evaluating HTLV-III Antibody Tests." *Lancet,* 1985.
  4. Mayer, K.H.; Stoddard, A.M.; et. al., "Human T-Lymphotropic Virus Type III in High-Risk, Antibody-Negative Homosexual Men." *Annals of Internal Medicine,* 1986.
  5. Kaplan, H.S.; Sager, J.J.; and Schiavi, R.C., "AIDS and the Sex Therapist." *Journal of Sex and Marital Therapy,* Winter 1985.
  6. Ulstrup, J.C.; Skaug, K.; et. al., "Sensitivity of Western Blotting (Compared with ELISA and Immunofluorescence) During Seroconversion After HTLV-III Infection." *Lancet,* 1986.
  7. Ward, J.W.; Grindon A.J.; et. al., "Laboratory and Epidemiologic Evaluation of an Enzyme Immunoassay for Antibodies to HTLV-III." *Journal of the American Medical Association,* 1986.
  8. Crenshaw, T.L., *Condom Advertisements.* Testimony Before the House Subcommittee on Health and the Environment, February 10, 1987.
  9. Marmor, M., "Why Patients Should Be Tested." *Journal of the American Medical Association,* 1987.
 10. Marmor, M., Letter to *The New York Times,* May 23, 1987.
 11. Goldert, J.J., "What Is Safe Sex? Suggested Standards Linked to Testing for the Human Immunodeficiency Virus." *New England Journal of Medicine,* 1987.
 12. Crenshaw, T.L., *AASECT Guidelines for AIDS Counseling,* 1987.
 13. Francis, D.P., and Chin, J., "The Prevention of Acquired Immunodeficiency in the U.S.—An Objective Strategy for Medicine, Public Health, Business, and the Community." *Journal of the American Medical Association,* 1987.

V. *AIDS the Disease*
  1. Soundbend, J., et al., "Acquired Immunodeficiency Syndrome, Opportunistic Infections and Malignancies in Male Homosexuals." *Journal of the American Medical Association,* 1983.

2. *Focus on AIDS: A Clinical Appraisal.* Proceeding of symposium on AIDS. Mérieux Institute, Inc., 1984.
3. Kanki, P.J., et al., "New Human T-Lymphotropic Retrovirus Related to Similar T-Lymphotropic Virus Type III." *Science,* 1985.
4. Schaad, U.B., et al., "Acquired Immunodeficiency Syndrome (AIDS) in Pediatric Patients." *Helv. Paediat. Acta.,* 1985.
5. *AIDS: Etiology, Diagnosis, Treatment and Prevention,* DeVit, V.T., Hellman, S., and Rosenberg, S.A., editors. Lippincot, 1986.
6. *AIDS: Facts and Issues,* Gong, V. and Rudnick, N., editors. Rutgers University Press, 1986.
7. Centers for Disease Control, "Classification System for Human T-Lymphotropic Virus Type III/Lymphadenopathy-Associated Virus Infections." *Morbidity and Mortality Weekly Reports,* May 1986.
8. Altman, L.K., "Data Suggests AIDS Risk Rises Yearly After Infection." *The New York Times,* March 3, 1987.
9. "AIDS: Statistics But Few Answers:" Report on the Third International Conference on AIDS. Washington D.C., June 1–5, 1987. *Science,* June 12, 1987.

VI. *Heterosexual Transmission of AIDS*

1. Redfield, R.R., et al., "Frequent Transmission of HTLV-III Among Spouses of Patients with AIDS-Related Complex and AIDS." *Journal of the American Medical Association,* 1985.
2. Kreiss, J.K., et al., "Antibody to Human-T Lymphotropic Virus Type III in Wives of Hemophiliacs." *Annals of Internal Medicine,* 1985.
3. Luzi, G., et al. "Transmission of HTLV-III Infection by Heterosexual Contact." *Lancet,* 1985.
4. Marmor, M., et al., "Possible Female-to-Female Transmission of HIV." *Annals of Internal Medicine,* 1986.
5. Calebrese, L.H. and Gopalakvisha, K.V., "Transmission of HTLV-III from Man to Woman to Man."
6. Fischl, M.A., Dickerson, G.M., et al. "Evaluation of Heterosexual Partners, Children, and Household Contacts of Adults with AIDS." *Journal of the American Medical Association,* February 1987.
7. Update of the above-cited study Personal communication with the authors, June 1987.
8. Quinn, T.C., "AIDS in Africa: Evidence for Heterosexual Transmission of the Human Immunodeficiency Virus." *New York State Journal of Medicine,* May 1987.

9. Winkelstein, W., et al., "Sexual Practices and Risks of Infection by HIV." *Journal of the American Medical Association*, 1987.
10. Des Jarlais, D.C., et al., "Intravenous Drug Use and the Heterosexual Transmission of the HIV: Current Trends in New York City." *New York State Journal of Medicine*, May 1987.
11. Steigbigel, N.H., et al., "Heterosexual Transmission of Infection and Disease by the Human Immunodeficiency Virus (HIV)." *III International Conference on AIDS*, Washington, D.C., June 1987.

VII. *Transmission of AIDS by Infected Blood.*
1. Centers for Disease Control, "Acquired Immunodeficiency Syndrome (AIDS): Precautions for Clinical and Laboratory Staffs." *Morbidity and Mortality Weekly Reports*, 1982.
2. Centers for Disease Control, "Recommendations to Decrease the Risk of Transmitting Infectious Diseases from Blood Donors," *Food and Drug Administration*, 1983.
3. Curron, J.W., "Acquired Immunodeficiency Syndrome (AIDS) Associated With Transfusions." *New England Journal of Medicine*, 1984.
4. Centers for Disease Control, "Provisional Public Health Service Inter-Agency Recommendations for Screening Donated Blood and Plasma for Antibodies to the Virus Causing Acquired Immunodeficiency Syndrome." *Morbidity and Mortality Weekly Reports*, 1985.
5. Schorr, J.B., et al., "Prevalence of HTLV-III Antibody in American Blood Donors." *New England Journal of Medicine*, 1985.
6. *AIDS Update*, National Hemophilia Foundation, 1985.
7. "Revised Definition of High-Risk Groups with Respect to Acquired Immunodeficiency Syndrome (AIDS)." *Food and Drug Administration*, 1985.
8. Kingsley, L.A., et al., "Risk Factors for Seroconversion to HIV Among Male Homosexuals." *Lancet*, 1987.

VIII. *Sex Therapy and Sexology*
1. Kinsey, A.C., et al., *Sexual Behavior in the Human Male.* Saunders, 1948.
2. Masters, W.H., and Johnson, V., *Human Sexual Inadequacy.* Little Brown, 1970.
3. ———, *Homosexuality in Perspective*, Little Brown, 1979
4. Kaplan, H.S., *The New Sex Therapy*, Bruner Mazel, 1974.
5. ———, *Disorders of Sexual Desire*, Bruner Mazel, 1979.
6. ——— (with D.F. Klein), *Sexual Aversion, Sexual Phobias, and Panic Disorders.* Bruner Mazel, 1987.

About the Author

HELEN SINGER KAPLAN received her Ph.D. from Columbia University where she conducted research on the interaction between drugs and learning, and she holds an M.D. from the New York Medical College. She has a background of learning theory, psychosomatic medicine, and psychoanalysis. Dr. Kaplan was a recipient of an NIH Career Teaching Grant and was Director of the Psychosomatic Service at Metropolitan Hospital.

Her interest in sexual disorders began when she worked with disadvantaged women at the Metropolitan Hospital in New York City in the psychosomatic-GYN clinic which she organized in 1965. Since that time her contributions to sexual medicine have been many and important.

Dr. Kaplan has integrated the behavioral sex therapy methods of Masters and Johnson with brief psychodynamic treatment for resolving underlying emotional and marital problems. Her work in separating the orgasm, excitement, and desire phases of the human sexual response was adopted by the American Psychiatric Association, and by the World Health Organization as the basis for the modern classification of sexual disorders in 1980.

Among her pioneering books is *The New Sex Therapy*, which has become a standard textbook for the treatment of sexual disorders throughout the world and has been translated into eleven languages. She was the first to recognize the syndrome of *disorders of sexual desire*, and published a book with that title in 1979. Dr. Kaplan has brought together the medical and psychological aspects of sexual medicine in a text, *The Evaluation of Sexual Disorders: Psychological and Medical Aspects*, in 1983. She has recently finished a book describing her new method of treating patients who suffer from *sexual aversion phobias and panic disorders* with a combination of antipanic medication and psychosexual therapy. She is currently continuing to pursue her interest in integrating the physical and mental elements of sexual disorders and is now working on a guide entitled *Medical Screening of Sexual Disorders* for physicians and sexual healthcare professionals.

In 1970 she founded, and now heads, the first Human Sexuality Program within a medical institution, at the New York Hospital–Cornell Medical Center. This program is involved both in research and patient care and is also responsible for teaching human sexuality to medical students and residents. It also provides advanced training for professionals from all over the world in the diagnosis and treatment of sexual disorders.

In addition to her academic work, Dr. Kaplan heads a private practice group for the treatment and evaluation of sexual disorders in New York City.

She has long been interested in sex education and has lectured widely here and abroad, and she writes a monthly column on sexual medicine for *Redbook* magazine.

Dr. Kaplan's husband encouraged the writing of this book because of his deep concern for the welfare of children. She has three children: Dr. Phillip Kaplan, who was extremely helpful in critiquing the scientific validity of the biological aspects of the book; Dr. Peter Kaplan, who lent his energetic support for this project; and a daughter, Jennifer, to whom this book is dedicated and who is following her stepfather in pursuing a business career.

This is the first book Dr. Kaplan has written for the general public. She was compelled to do so because of her deep concern for women everywhere — and for their partners — and for their children whose lives are being held hostage by the threat of AIDS.